Aphrodisiac
Foods

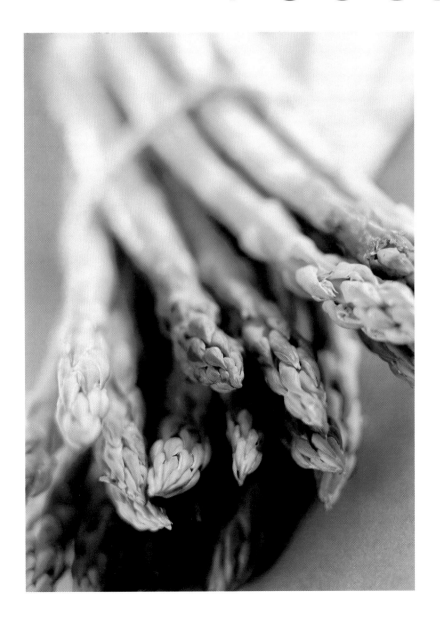

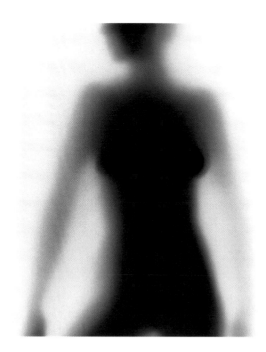

THIS IS A CARLTON BOOK

Text and Design © Carlton Books Limited, 1999

This edition published by Carlton Books Limited, 1999

A CIP catalogue record for this book is available from the British Library

ISBN 1 85868 713 6

Project editor: Camilla MacWhannell
Project art direction: Zoë Mercer
Design and Editorial: Joanne Dovey and Neil Williams
Production: Alexia Turner
Picture Research: Alex Pepper
Special photography: Howard Shooter

Printed and bound in Italy

PICTURE ACKNOWLEDGEMENTS

The publishers would like to thank the following sources for their kind permission to reproduce the pictures in this book:

AKG London 6, 84t/Erich Lessing 59, 88
Bridgeman Art Library, London/New York/Laing Art Gallery, Newcastle-upon-Tyne, *Isabella and the Pot of Basil, 1867 by William Holman Hunt (1827–1910)* 73tl/Stapleton Collection, *Erotic Trio in fancy dress, illustration from The Pleasures of Eros, 1917 by Gerda Wegener (b.1889)* 7/Victoria & Albert Museum, London, *Lovers from the 'Poem of the Pillow' ('Uta makura') by Kittagawa Utamaro (1753–1806)* 49
Cephas Christine Fleurent 33/Vince Hart 41/Diana Mewes 83, 86b, 93/Alain Proust 43, 51
Stockfood 32, 42, 46, 48, 58, 61, 63
TOP Herve Amiard 37, 39, 56/Daniel Czap 64/Pierre Hussenot 44, 62/J.F.Riviere 54/Ryman/Cabannes 65/Manfred Seelow 47/ Tripelon/ Jarry 31
et archive 14br, 36, 55
Iain McKell 92
Howard Shooter 1, 3, 10, 11, 12, 13, 19–28, 30, 50, 70, 71, 72, 73br, 74–78, 81, 84b, 85, 86t, 87, 89, 90, 94, 95
Tony Stone Images Donna Day 91/Chris Everard 67/ Carol Ford 38/Bruce Forster 4/Ian O'Leary 14t/Kevin Summers 15

Every effort has been made to acknowledge correctly and contact the source and/copyright holder of each picture, and Carlton Books Limited apologises for any unintentional errors or omissions which will be corrected in future editions of this book.

Aphrodisiac Foods

Eat Your Way to Ecstasy

HILARY JOHNSTONE
CRAIG DODD

CARLTON

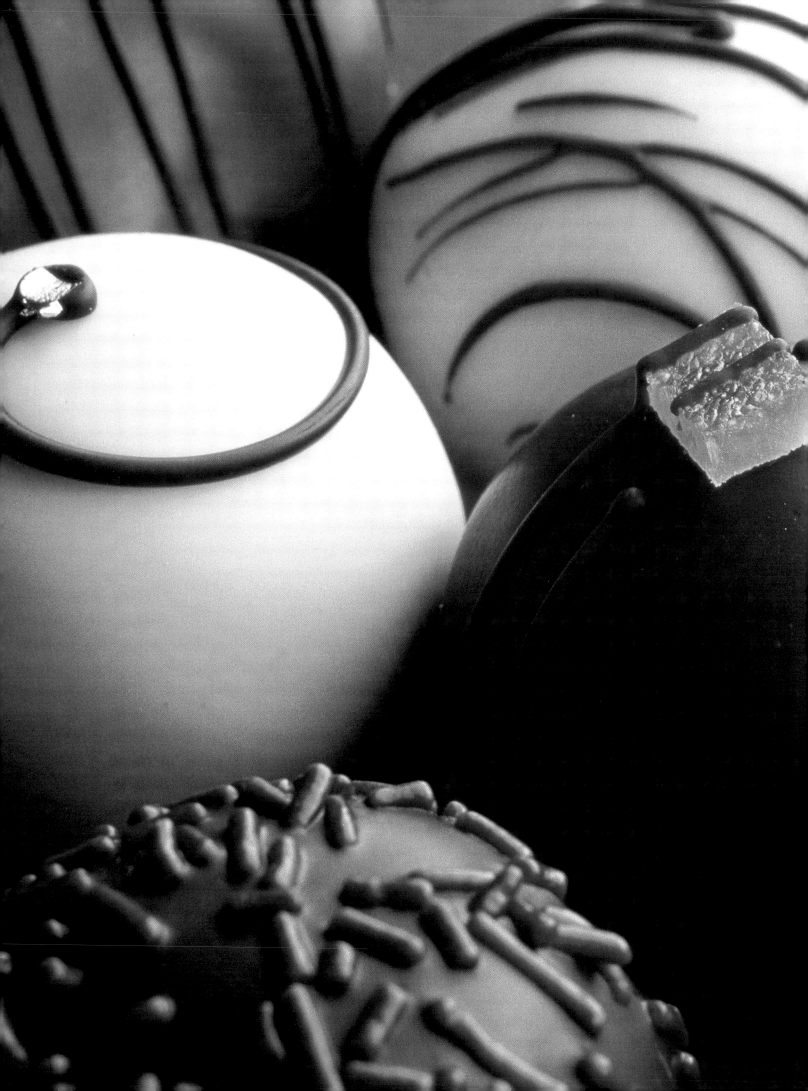

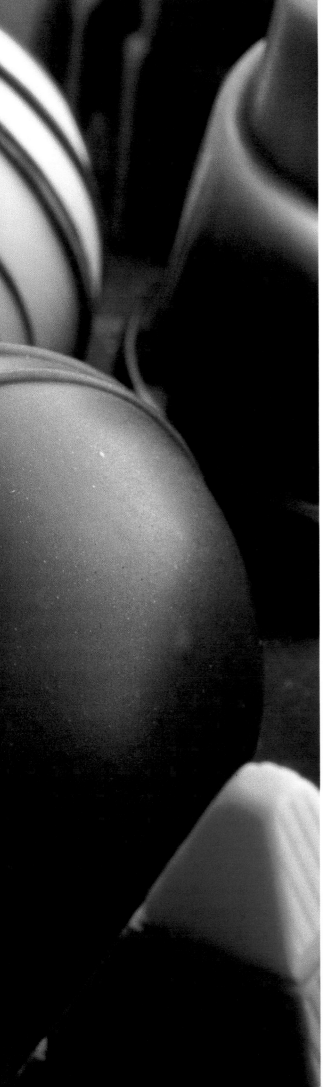

CONTENTS

Introduction

Bat's blood, rhino horn, goat's testicles, magpie excrement and dead kites are but a few of the odious ingredients used by the ancients in their search for aphrodisiac potions to enhance their sexual performance. So desperate was their search, they did not realise they were dicing with death as they happily drank possets laced with sulphur and red arsenic, or consumed the dreaded Spanish Fly, the powdered remains of a beetle from southern Europe, capable of driving people mad – and not through desire.

WORKS SUCH AS THE *KAMA SUTRA* PROMOTED APHRODISIACAL FOOD TO ENHANCE SEXUAL PERFORMANCE.

Some of the ancient potions will feature in this book, but only those still relevant today, or to underline how old beliefs can turn into modern practices. Most of these come from the few extant sources.

One of the earliest sources, and easily the most famous, is the Hindu *Kama Sutra*, written between the first and fourth centuries AD. Roughly contemporaneous was Pliny the Elder, whose major work, *Natural History*, attempts to define all living creatures and their

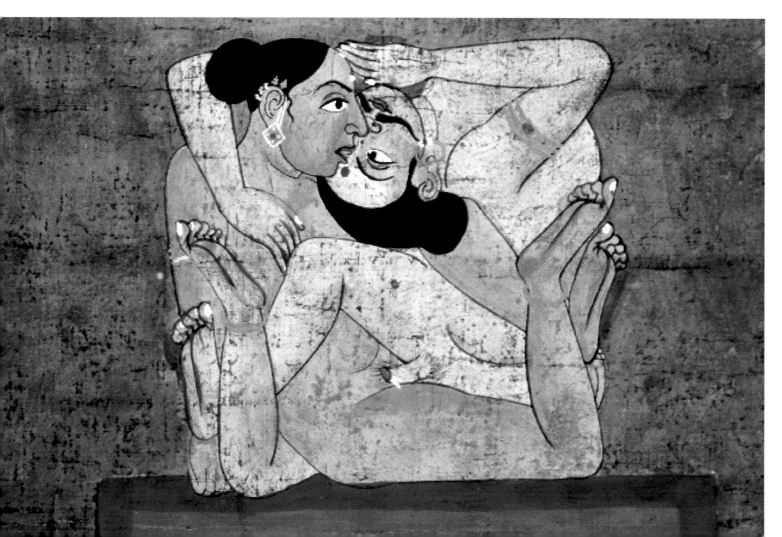

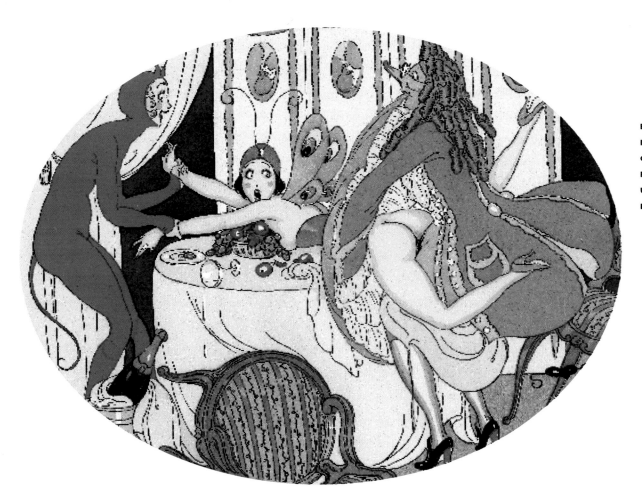

behaviour. No explanation of aphrodisiac properties could ever be too far-fetched for him.

Shaik al-Nefwazi wrote *The Perfumed Garden* in the 16th century, gathering together all the sexual lore of Araby. He had an altogether more straightforward approach. Other writers include the Greek, Galen, a first century army doctor, Dioscorides, and several Roman sources. A slightly more scientific approach was taken by Culpeper in his *Herbal*, published in the early 18th century.

In many cultures there were variations on two basic rules defining what an aphrodisiac is. The first was the Law of Similarity, sometimes referred to as the Doctrine of Signatures. This laid down that the shape of a plant or animal dictated its properties. Needless to say, the shape was often reminiscent of genitalia, male and female. The main examples are the two roots which resemble the whole human body, Mandrake and Ginseng. Mandrake was reputed to scream when pulled out of the ground, before being turned into a charm. Ginseng on the other hand was ascribed, and still is, remarkable powers. Sir Edwin Arnold wrote in his *Travels* that 'The Korean people believe that it is a complete panacea for all mortal ills, mental and physical... and fills the heart with hilarity and adds a decade to the span of life'. He

might also have added that many people believed firmly that it was the best food to increase an already healthy sexual appetite. It can be used in various dishes, but loses some efficacy in cooking. It can also be taken straight as capsules or pills.

The second law defining aphrodisiacs is the Rule of Rarity, which is self-explanatory. Many vegetables, herbs and spices which are commonplace now, were once rarities imported from afar. This gave them a certain allure and they were attributed special properties.

The foods in this book belong very much to today, but how their properties were first ascribed lies in the mists of history. We have more knowledge than the ancients, as we know the importance of balanced diets and the quality of the food we eat, but still there is the tantalising thought at the back of every mind that there might just be that one dish, that one spice, that one ingredient that may enhance sexual performance.

This book does not offer the instant gratification of a drug such as Viagra. It is more a gentle guide to those foods which help consistently over a long period of time. It is also for those who think that food and wine should be erotic and exotic, sexual and sensual.

Note: The recipes included are general guides. Specific recipes are readily found in many cookbooks.

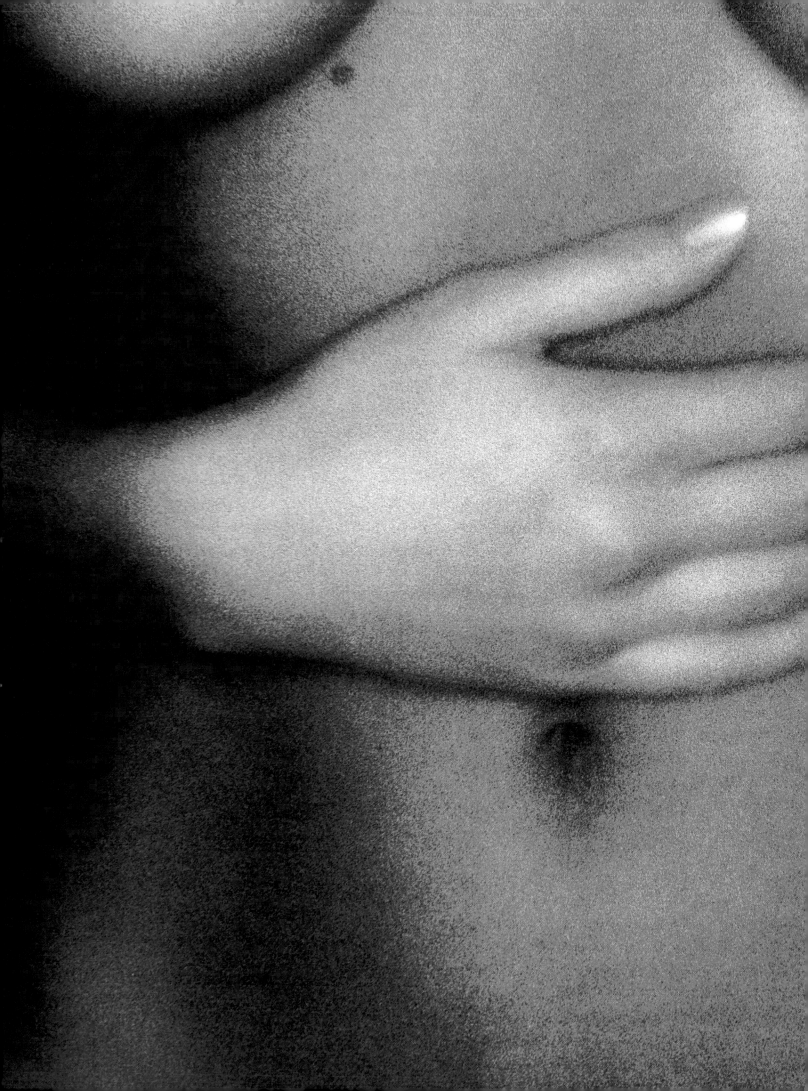

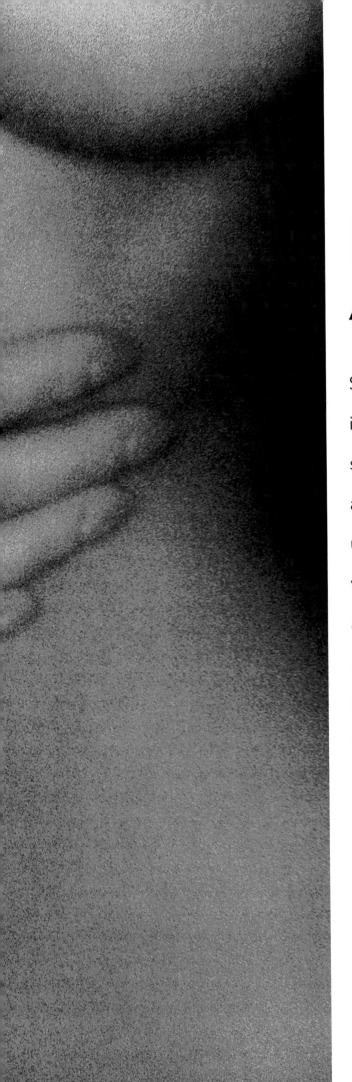

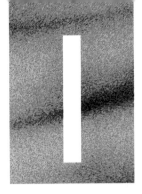

FOREPLAY
AND AFTERPLAY

Setting the scene for an aphrodisiac meal is of vital importance. Anticipation is of the essence, as is the stimulation of the olfactory and visual senses. Table settings are crucial, and need not be in the classical style. In fact, an unusual arrangement might add to the anticipation. A table without cutlery will immediately suggest a hands-on approach, and there are few more suggestive ways of eating than with the fingers. Lifting asparagus spears to the lips, as they drip with melted butter... tearing apart some innocent crustacean, before gnawing at the succulent flesh... breaking apart an artichoke, before scraping off the flesh with bared teeth... manhandling a fig... dipping strawberries in champagne, before biting into the sensual berry...

Creating the setting

Floral decorations add both visual and olfactory delights. A formal bouquet or designer piece may be off-putting, unless it is for an evening dress and black tie affair. On the other hand a simple scattering of rose petals (some prefer the heads of miniature roses) or something more adventurous, such as orange blossom, marigold petals or bright nasturtium flowers can be very effective. The latter can also be nibbled throughout the meal, the spicy nasturtium taste being particularly inflaming. If you do not wish to use them as decoration, put them in your salad bowl.

If you must have a formal decoration, use orchids or some similarly suggestive looking bloom. And if your budget runs to it float a few gardenias in an attractive bowl, alongside some scented candles. Rose petals also work well.

Other seasonal perfumes to use, if they are available, include honeysuckle, which tickles the senses, and jasmine which lulls them.

OPPOSITE: CANDLELIGHT ENHANCES BOTH FOOD AND DINERS.

BELOW: ROSE PETALS HAVE A TIMELESS ALLURE.

If fresh foliage is not readily available, deploy scented candles to create a visual element. Too easily discarded as a cliché, candlelight still provides the most magical, flickering surroundings for an erotic meal. Everyone looks good in candlelight and any slight blunders in the food department are visually masked. The range of perfumed candles available today ensures that there is something right for every occasion.

Appetisers

Having created the setting, make sure that your pre-meal nibbles, with a suggestive aperitif of your choice, do nothing to detract from what is to follow. Nuts can be most effective.

Many nuts have long been considered to have aphrodisiac qualities. You do not have to go to the excesses of the ancients. Nefwazi, in *The Perfumed Garden*, suggests that virility can be enhanced by '...eating twenty almonds and one hundred grains of the pine tree' before bedtime, for three successive days. This concoction was also promoted by Galen.

Pine nuts have long had a reputation as an aphrodisiac, especially around the Mediterranean, as well as in the East. One of the first cookery writers, Apicus, suggests in his cookbook *De re coquinaria* that '...a concoction of pine seeds, cooked onions, white mustard and pepper is most effective.' The Roman poet, Ovid, also includes 'the nuts that the sharp-leaved pine brings forth' in his book, *The Art of Love*.

There are seven varieties of pine nut to choose from, but the most commonly available are the seeds of the Italian stone pine and the Swiss stone pine. In America, the seeds of the Mexican pine nut are more readily available. However, if you can find them, the most effective pine nuts come from the Chilgoza Pine which grows in the northwestern Himalayas, at around 3000 metres above sea level. They are a staple food for the inhabitants of the Kunawar region, noted for their prodigious birthrate. Sadly, political instability in the region, between Afghanistan and Tibet, has limited supplies reaching the West. Crushed pine nuts can also be used to make an aphrodisiac starter, a soup with a vegetable or chicken base. Also the nuts can be mashed with

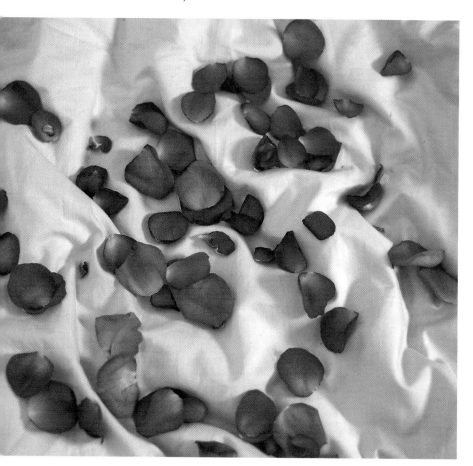

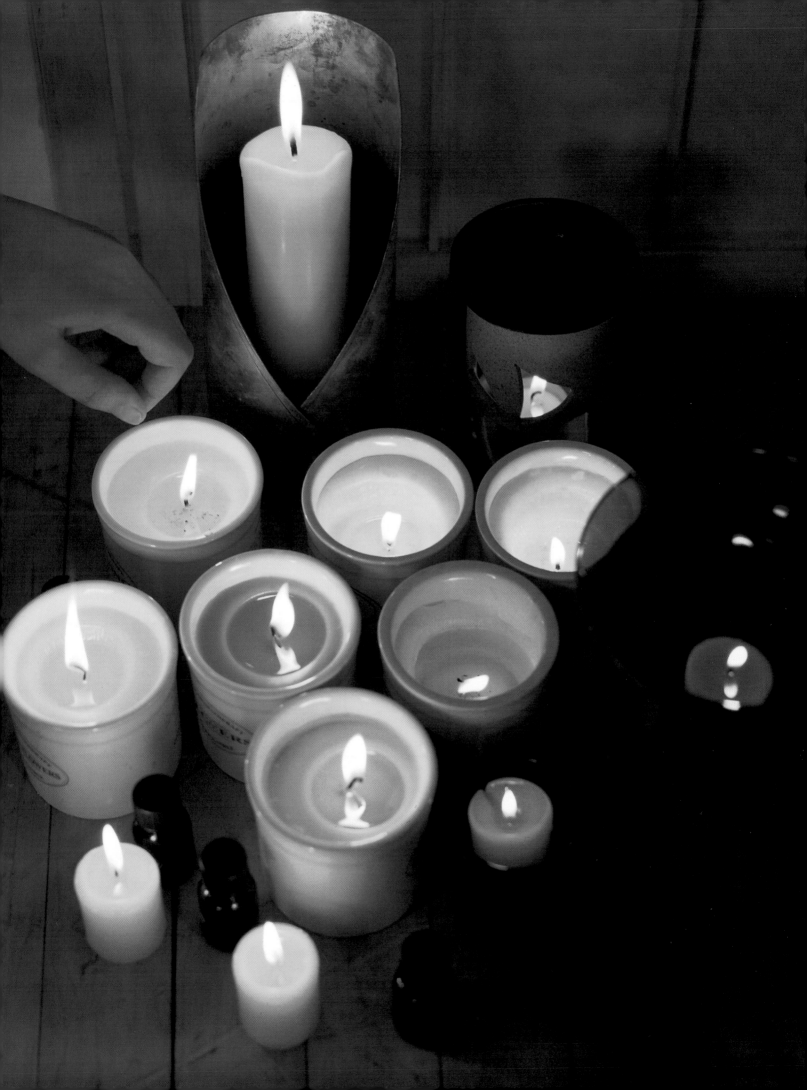

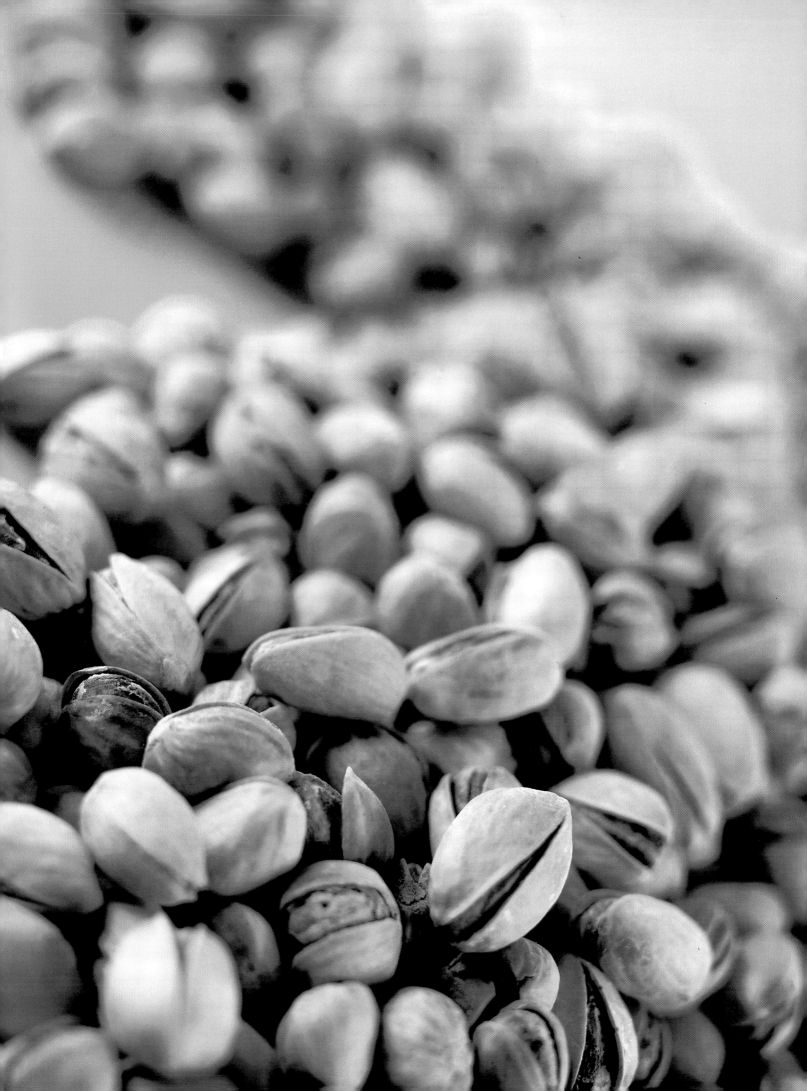

prawns and paprika (to taste) to make a spicy spread. Or they can be roasted to add to a dish of spicy mussels. On an evening out take a pack of roasted pine nuts to the cinema to enhance the effect of a romantic movie.

Almonds, with their highly evocative aroma, have always been prized in both the Near and Far East. If you can find fresh nuts and then manage to crack them, roast your own. Most are available ready dried and roasted to be added to your nut bowl or made into a soup. Poach a pound of nuts until soft, then blend them with three hard-boiled egg yolks. Add a half-litre (approximately a pint) of chicken stock and then a dash of cream. Heat gently, in a double-boiler if possible. Actual quantities of liquid may vary according to whether the nuts are fresh or dried. Adjust to suit your style, your taste and the occasion.

Pistachio nuts are a joy eaten plain, but can also be ground to a paste to be added to both spicy and sweet dishes. Just thinking about pistachio ice cream can be erotic. Create a simple pistachio soup based on those in many Arabic erotic manuals, for the Arabs believed in the power of pistachio. Simply blanche them, make a paste and add to a soup stock of your choice. They can also be used to garnish simple starters involving other ingredients with aphrodisiac properties, such as apricots. Take fresh or rehydrated apricots. Split part through and fill with goat's cheese mixed with crushed pistachio nuts. Bake in a medium oven until soft. Allow to cool and sprinkle generously with more crushed nuts. Excess is everything.

Walnuts feature in many ancient manuals, and were used by the Romans in fertility rites. They were thrown, as we throw rice, at wedding ceremonies to encourage fecundity. They are effective eaten plain, or made into a simple soup with the emperor of aphrodisiacs, garlic. Pound fresh walnuts and garlic to taste and add to chicken stock. If dried walnuts are used, add liquid to achieve the consistency you like.

The high protein content of all nuts accounts for their invigorating qualities which, in the long run, will help prolong and enhance sexual activity. To enhance the power of nuts, add a scattering of sunflower seeds to your nut bowl. Whether raw or incorporated in a

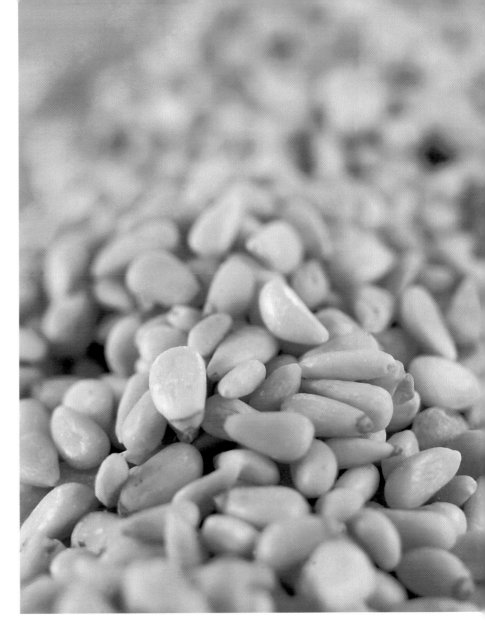

cooked dish, they have always been considered high on the aphrodisiac register.

After your initial nibbles enjoy your aphrodisiac meal, but have no nagging doubts about how it will end.

Endgame

Essential will be good quality coffee. Instant coffee will produce the result the very name suggests. Caffeine stimulates, which is why some sects such as the Mormons do not drink it (they then go on to have enormous families – perhaps they are trying to tell us something!). In the Middle East, home of aphrodisiamania, coffee is almost a second religion. In America, coffee has also created a cult with a language of its own, though in this case it is distinctly non-aphrodisiac. Who could be turned on when their partner orders a 'half-caf, double-tall, non-fat, whole-milk foam, bone-dry, half-pump mocha, half raw sug, double lid, capp, to fly', as supermodel stereotypes do? She just wants a large, not-too-frothy, mocha-blend

ABOVE: PINE NUTS ARE UNIVERSALLY REGARDED AS AN APHRODISIAC.

OPPOSITE: PISTACHIO NUTS CAN BE TAKEN PLAIN OR AS AN INGREDIENT OF SOUP OR ICE CREAM.

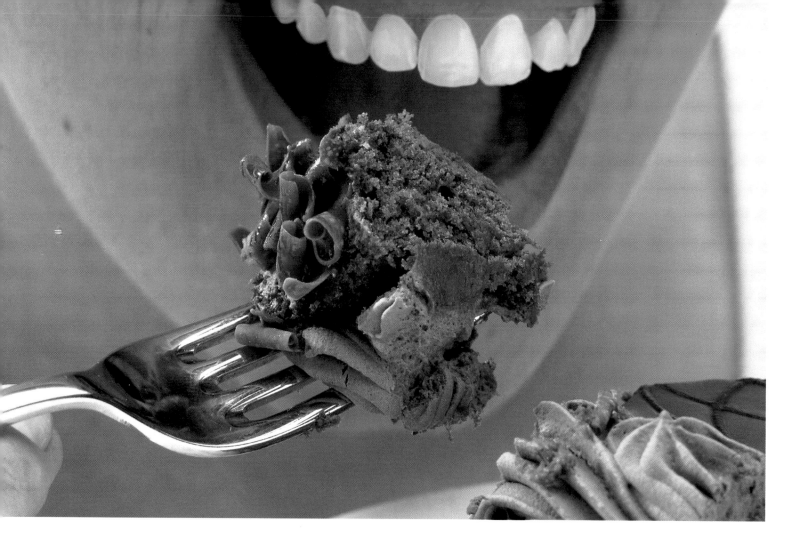

cappuccino, caffeine reduced, to take away. Stick to heavily aromatic pure arabica coffee, with a dash of your favourite liqueur to add body, aroma and lust. And perhaps a dusting of cinnamon for heat.

And as a complement to the coffee? Chocolate, chocolate and more chocolate. Some believe that chocolate is even better than sex. It is one of the few aphrodisiacs that can be scientifically proved to have constituents which stimulate certain areas of the brain, but that is to dampen the romance. Thank the Aztecs for discovering it (perhaps it encouraged their excesses) and the Spanish conquistadors for bringing it back to Europe. Not for nothing are the greatest chocolates – truffles of whatever flavour – named after the greatest vegetable aphrodisiac. Allied with champagne or certain spices, the combination can be overpowering. At the end of an aphrodisiac meal perhaps restraint is called for in the chocolate department, if the ultimate aim of the evening is to be achieved. Go for high cocoa solid content, but small amounts. A little Belgian creation can go a long way.

Chocolate is notoriously difficult with alcohol, but experiment with highly aromatic dessert wines. You do not have to go to the excesses of Chateau d'Yquem,

which might cause mental anguish when the bill is presented, but there are now many other heady flavours, available by the half-bottle, where the 'nose', or smell alone, causes palpitations.

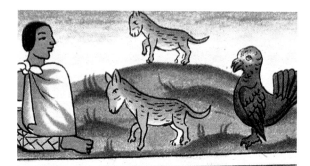

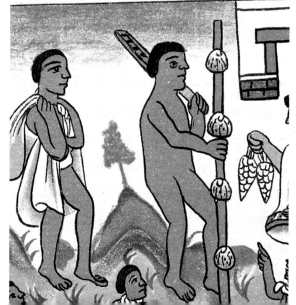

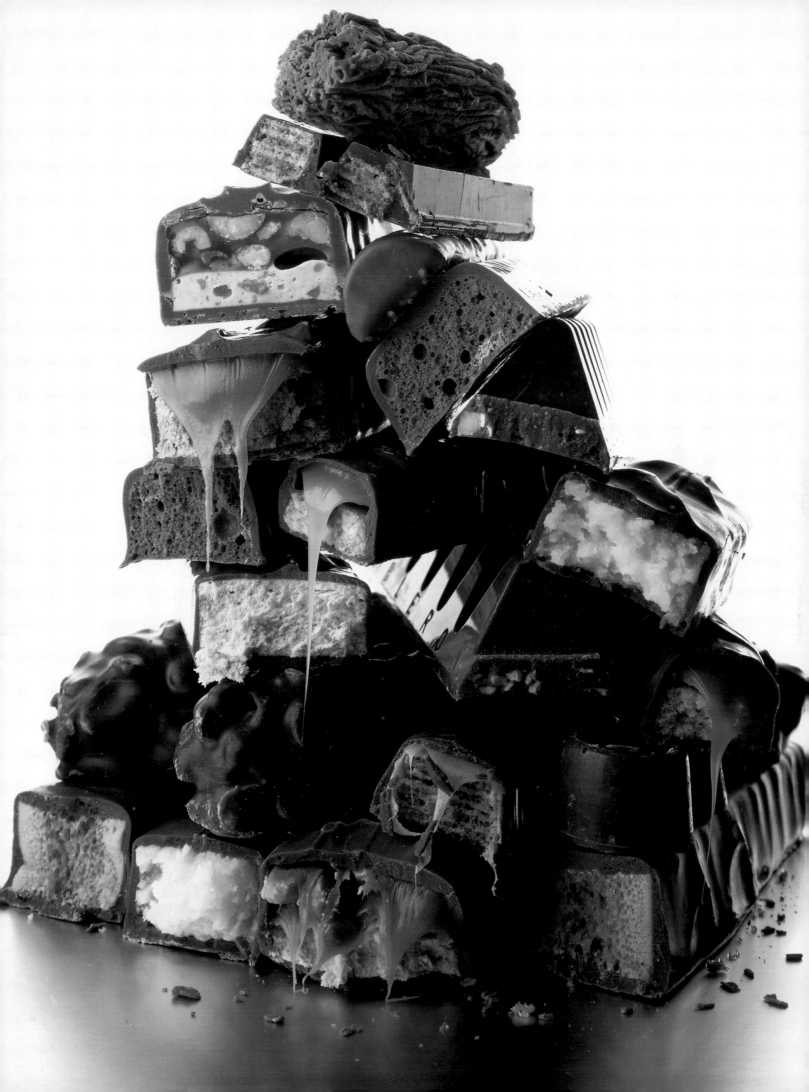

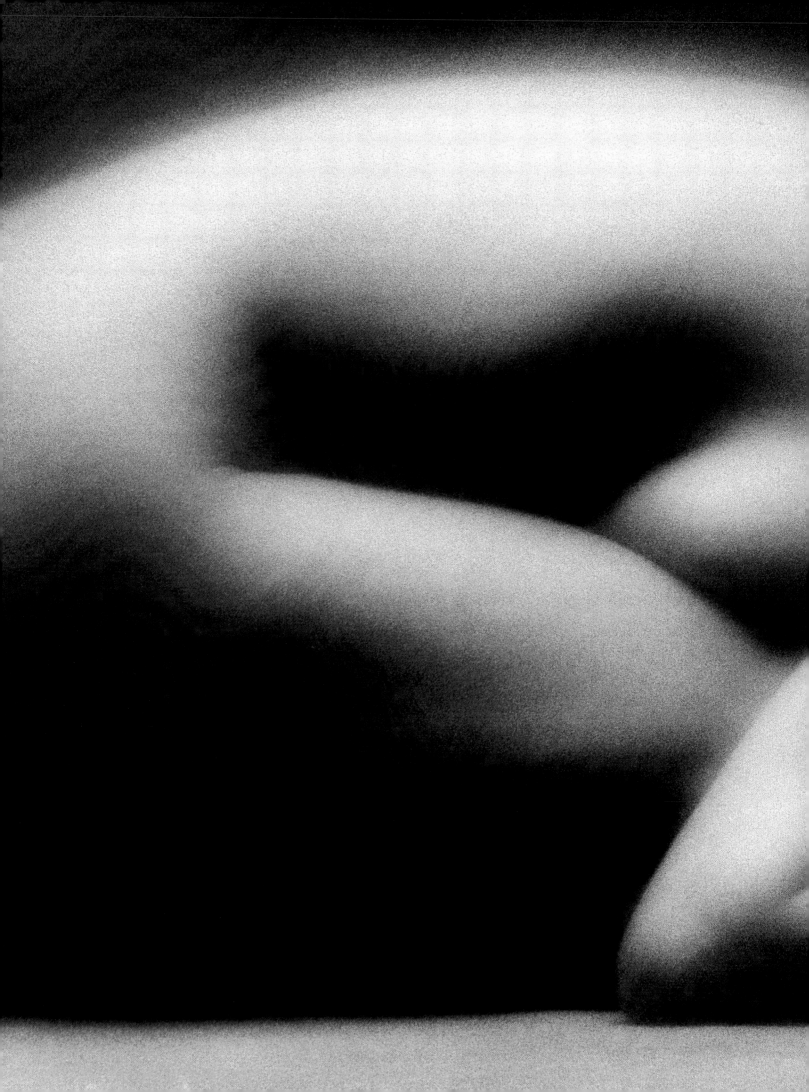

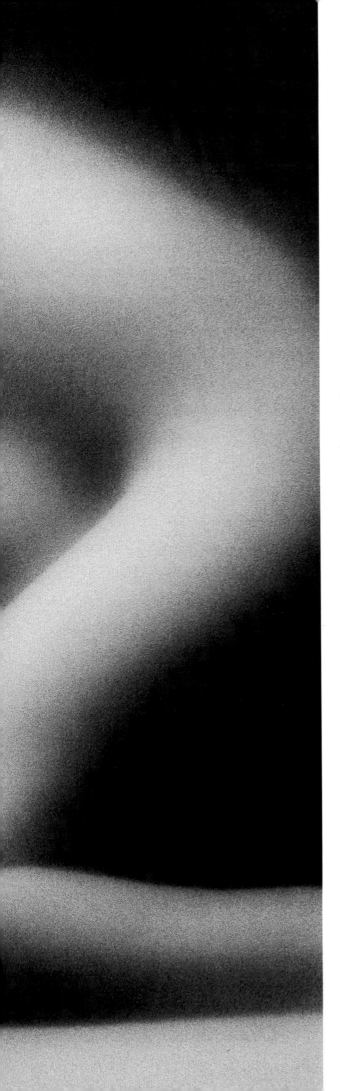

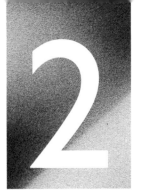

NATURE'S GARDEN OF APHRODISIA

There is a whole cornucopia of vegetable aphrodisiacs, most having gained their reputation back in ancient times. Some can be presented as simple vegetable dishes, others can be powdered or liquidised for medicinal uses. In general, aphrodisiacs are most effective when taken in moderation, though the Marquis de Sade in his *120 Days of Sodom* wrote that the most potent erotic dinner should start with a bisque and then go on to twenty hors d'oeuvres, twenty entrées, twenty poultry dishes, garnished game, ornamental roasts, pastries hot and cold, desserts, hot-house fruits and ices. All of this should be washed down with three different Italian, Rhone and Rhine wines, two Greek wines and champagne!

**OPPOSITE: SENSUALLY
SHAPED AND COLOURED
AUBERGINES.**

Root vegetables

Amongst root and related vegetables (not in the strict botanical sense) first comes angelica. It is the crystallised root of that plant and is helpful in avoiding cardiac deficiencies. It was used in the nineteenth century to help ladies overcome frigidity. Today, it is found mostly as a decoration on luxury chocolates and patisserie, presumably to counter the effects of their richness.

Carrots were popular in Ancient Greece to prepare a 'philtron' to combat venereal disease. The Arabs ate them stewed in milk to accentuate sexual activity. It was even thought that they helped you see in the dark, a convenient aid during amorous encounters. Puréed with coriander they make an attractive addition to any meat dish, but particularly game.

Eryngo is not widely available today, but does exist under its common name, Sea Holly. It features

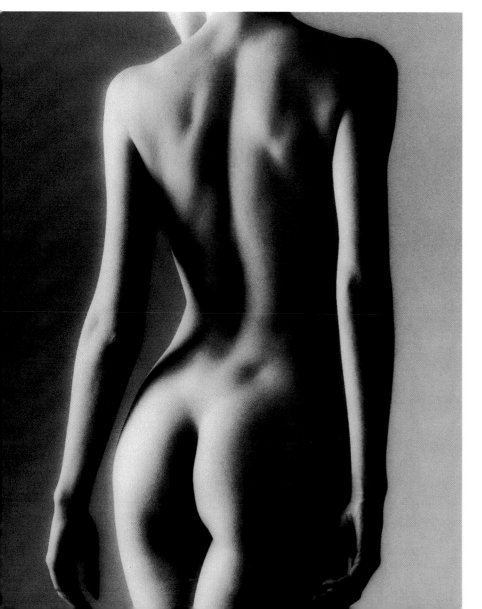

in Shakespeare's *Merry Wives of Windsor*, when Falstaff exclaims 'Hail kissing comfits and snow eringoes'. It has the appearance of a large thistle with blue flowers. The edible part is the fleshy root, which for centuries has been regarded as a powerful aphrodisiac. It was candied for consumption and used as a condiment. It was reputed to increase potency, and the Arabs found it an invigorating stimulant for both men and women. Dioscorides, a Greek army physician who lived in the first century AD, used it as an aid to digestion.

John Dryden, in his translation of the Roman satirist Juvenal, writes of the libertines:

*Who lewdly dancing at a midnight ball
For hot eryngoes and fat oysters call.*

Perhaps this particular aphrodisiac is due for a revival.

Potatoes were once highly regarded as an aphrodisiac, but as they became common, even universal, the aura of magic waned. Well into the seventeenth century they were valued and the Law of Rarity applied. When they were first introduced into Europe (by Thomas Heriot in England, not Sir Walter Raleigh, as in popular myth, and by Parmentier in France) they were highly prized. They were reputed to restore the vigour of aged gentlemen, which is why Falstaff also exclaimed to Mistress Quickly: 'Let the sky rain potatoes...'

Another esoteric root is mallow, which you can search for in marshy woodlands. If you are brave enough, pick it and use the root or squeeze the sap out of its stems. Pliny the Elder recommended the root cooked in goat's milk to enhance the sexual urge in men, whilst the sap, together with the root does much the same for women. If you are feeling over-amorous, the dry root will calm your urges.

Mediterranean vegetables

The Mediterranean family of vegetables is highly regarded. Aubergines are sensual to look at, with their glorious purple sheen and bulbous shape. In the history of aphrodisiacs they were used principally in the West Indies to make a paste with peppercorns, chives and pimentoes to be used as a genital excitant.

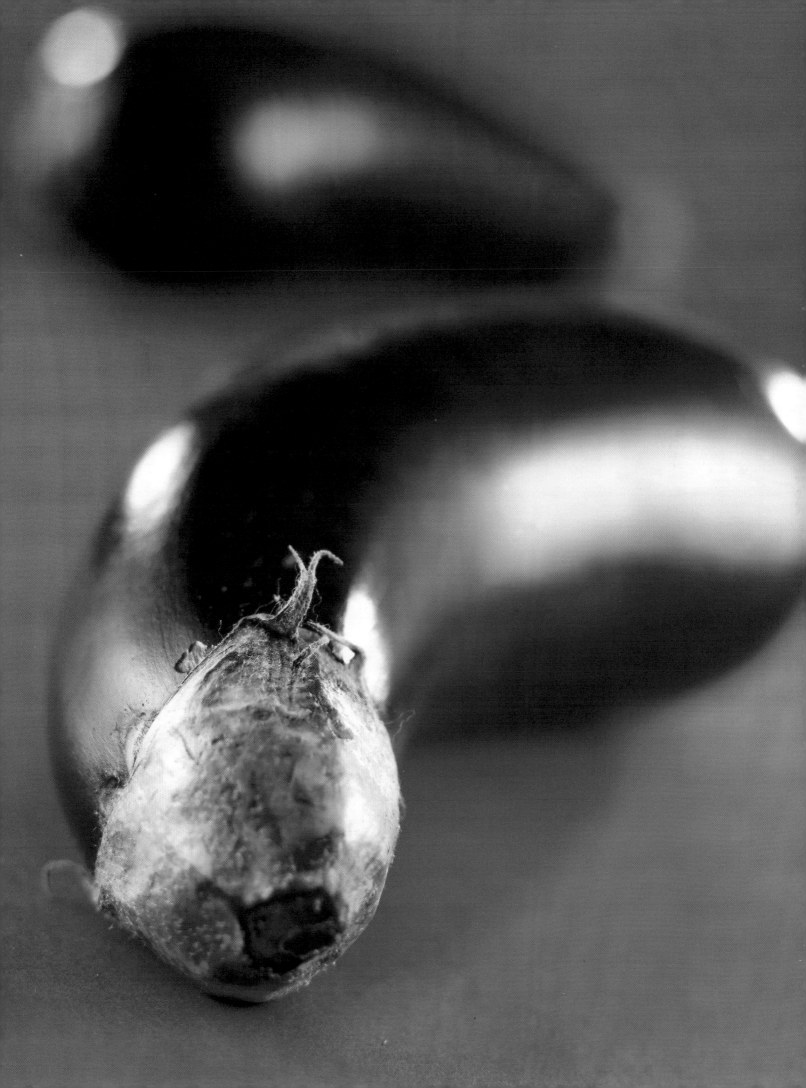

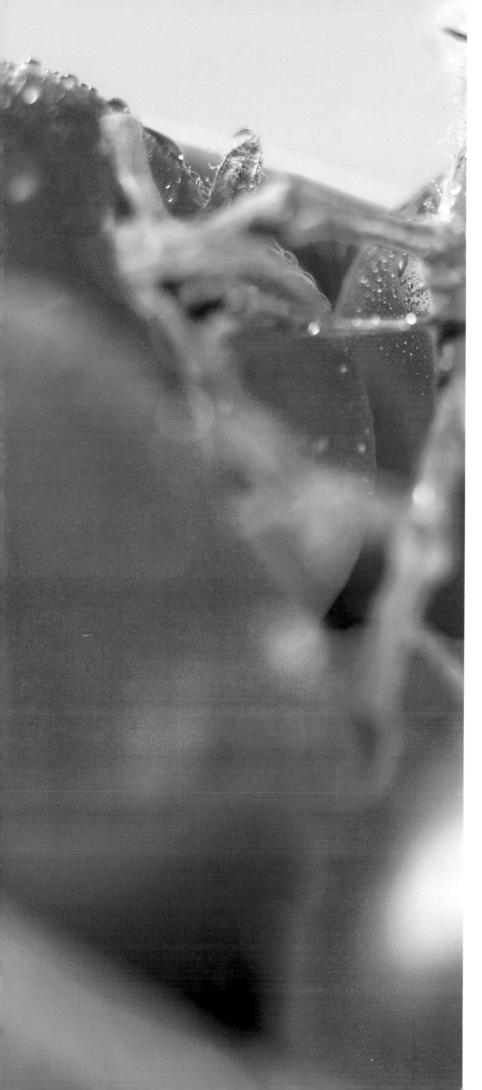

The Arabs took a more sensual approach and amongst their creations was the immortal Imam Bayaldi. The famed Imam fainted when the creation was put before him! Slice your aubergine lengthwise, keeping the stalk intact to help hold the dish together. Scoop out the flesh in big chunks and sprinkle with salt in a sieve to remove some water. The rest will be lost in the baking. Peel, de-seed and roughly chop some tomatoes. Mince some onion and garlic. Mix these ingredients together, add a pinch of ground cloves, seasoning to taste and a teaspoon of sugar. Fill the aubergine halves and bake for half an hour in a medium oven. You can vary the seasoning to suit yourself. Try sensual cinnamon sprinkled on top, or give it a hint of India with some cardamom or cumin seeds.

Tomatoes are now commonplace, but they enjoyed a considerable reputation when introduced to Europe from the New World. Only the seriously rich could afford them and, as the peasants watched their betters multiply prolifically, they ascribed this fecundity to their intake of this exotic fruit. Not only has the power of the tomato waned, but it has also become known that its romantic French name, 'pomme d'amour', actually has nothing to do with love, but is a mistranslation of the Italian 'pome de mori' – the apple of the Moors. Nevertheless, a good plum tomato, full of flavour, when allied to a creamy buffalo mozzarella cheese and fragrant basil, can produce a certain frisson.

Peppers, onions and mushrooms

Peppers feature mostly as aphrodisiacs when dried and powdered rather than as vegetables, but combined with aubergines, tomatoes, courgettes (which do not feature on the aphrodisiac scale due to their water content) and onions in a dish such as ratatouille, can offer some results. But perhaps this only works when eating it somewhere around the Mediterranean shores!

The onion family has a legendary reputation in the world of aphrodisia. Ovid rates them high, Martial advises that '...if your wife is old and your member

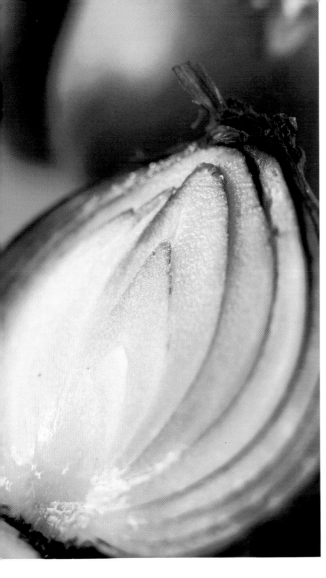

sexual activity has happened, but sadly it was all in the mind. But that is to underestimate the chanterelle, the oyster, the trompète de mort and their myriad relatives. If you are doing the picking yourself consult a guide. Most are edible, but the occasional puff-ball can cause trouble. A mixture of mushrooms, simply sautéed in a little butter, with a last-minute dash of oyster sauce, then piled onto a toasted brioche, provides a sensual feast of varying tastes and textures.

Beans

Beans were forbidden in nunneries under the rule of St. Jerome, who considered them sexually inflammatory. Broad beans have long been thought of as an aphrodisiac in Italy, while lentils played a similar part in the life of Ancient Greece. Broad beans are best young and fresh, lightly boiled and then stir-fried with diced bacon. Smoked bacon enhances their flavour.

exhausted, resort to the humble onion.' The onion's relationship with garlic enhances its power. Its culinary uses are legion and it can form the basis of many soups and stews, as well as standing on its own as a roasted vegetable or boiled and served with a simple white sauce. Traditional Arab use of the onion for sexual potency suggests boiling them with aromatic spices of your choice, then frying them with egg yolks. This dish should be eaten every day for a week.

The shallot, the onion's small sweet cousin, and the spring onion (scallion) were praised by Martial:

'If envious age relax the nuptial knot
Thy food be scallions, and thy feast shallot.'

Onion seed is the basis of many ancient remedies. Nefwazi recommends pounding them and mixing the powder with honey. Galen agreed.

Produce from the woods and fields include the whole mushroom family. The wild ones have been more praised for their hallucinatory powers than for their aphrodisiac gifts. They can convince that great

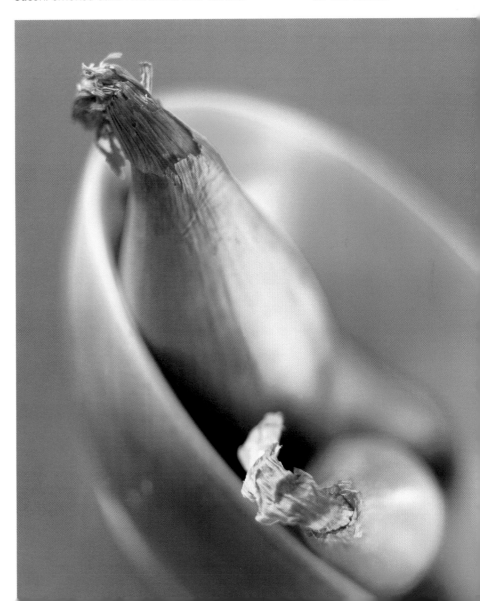

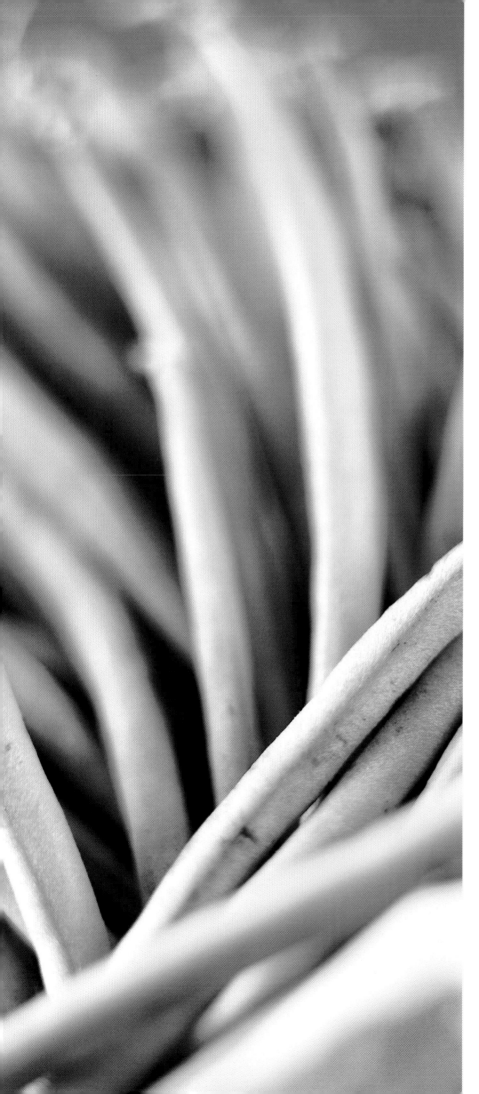

Lentils should be well-soaked and thoroughly cooked before being used in salads or as the basis for many other dishes. Simple ham hock, steamed, sat atop some lentils works particularly well.

Oriental vegetables

Bean sprouts are a staple of the oriental diet and as such were treasured by the poor who did not have access to the rarer foodstuffs available to their betters. To maximise their efficacy, freshness and quick cooking are essential. In proportions to suit your taste, take finely sliced red and green peppers, bamboo shoots, carrots, cucumber or courgette, together with chopped ginger, salt and pepper, a dash of dry sherry (or wine vinegar), soy sauce and chilli sauce (if preferred). Quickly stir-fry in sesame or other vegetable oil until softened, but still crisp. Add the bean sprouts and stir for a few minutes more. Add the soy sauce, sherry and chilli sauce at the very last minute for one quick stir. A variation, using much the same ingredients, is to turn them into a bean sprout salad. Simply add the raw ingredients to bean sprouts which have been boiled for 10 to 12 minutes. Mix together the sauce ingredients and pour over the salad.

Also from the Orient, bamboo shoots have been considered an aphrodisiac. The Chinese especially considered them effective. For reasons of availability tinned bamboo shoots can be used. They make an excellent accompaniment to bite-sized slivers of chicken, stir-fried with garlic, ginger and oyster sauce. Blanch the bamboo shoot slices and add to the stir-fry at the last minute or as a decorative garnish.

Chickpeas formed the basis of a popular stimulant for the Arabs. They were pounded to a paste with honey that had been heated with onion juice and a little added water. Taken before bedtime, particularly in winter, this concoction had an invigorating effect.

LEFT: EAT YOUR GREENS FOR ENJOYMENT.

RIGHT: LENTILS OF EVERY COLOUR FORM THE BASIS OF MANY APHRODISIACAL DISHES.

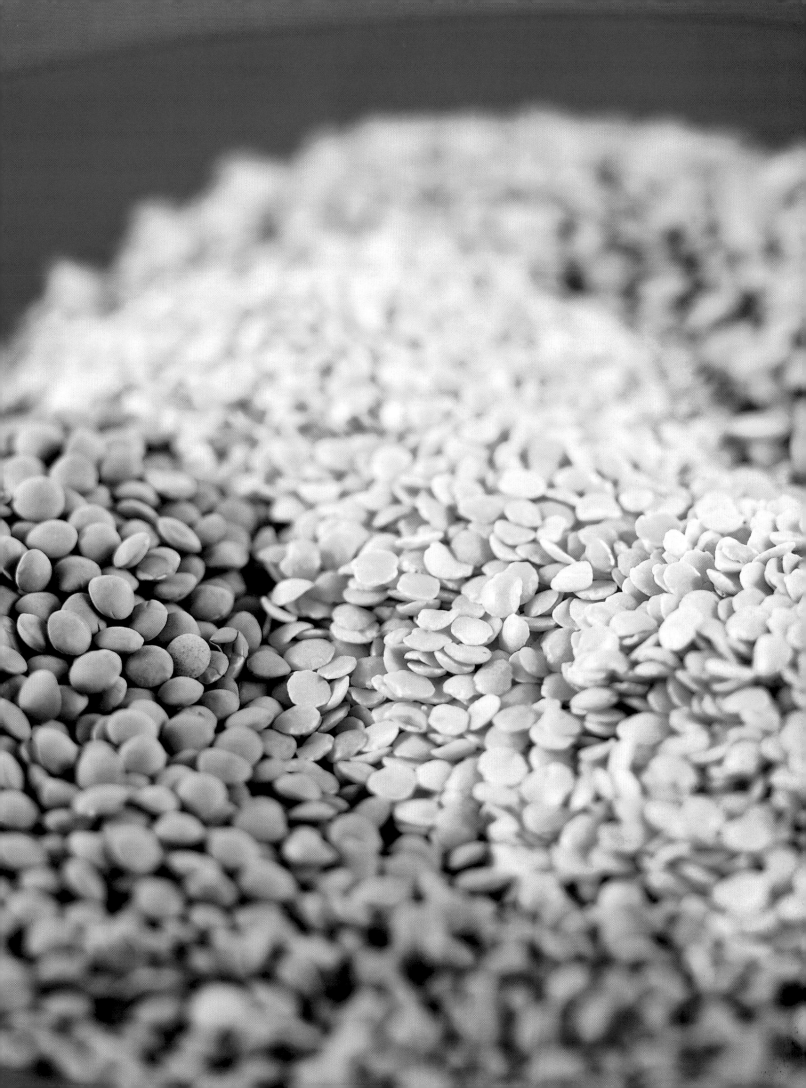

A variant of this dish is still popular today in the form of houmous; pounded chickpeas, with a little tahini (a sesame seed paste, not unlike peanut butter), olive oil and lemon juice. Serve with a swirl of olive oil, a sprinkling of paprika and some chopped parsley on top. The Ancient Romans knew a thing or two about chick peas. They fed them to their stallions.

Eat your greens

Freshly podded peas were also recommended by Nefwazi, though by few others. According to him, a dish which creates passion can be made by boiling peas briefly with onions, powdered cinnamon and crushed cardamom pods. Highly aromatic.

'Eat your greens' has become a familiar phrase. But it conceals a great truth. Cabbage sounds like the least attractive aphrodisiac, but it has been the base for many potions over the centuries. Crisp white cabbage, finely sliced and dressed with good mayonnaise and flavouring of choice, becomes coleslaw. Add some curry flavours for a more erotic taste. Cumin and turmeric are most effective, but you can use a spoon of ready-made curry paste of your choice. As with broad beans, finely sliced cabbage, stir-fried in sesame oil – or another favourite, flavoured vegetable oil – goes well with diced bacon.

The cabbage family includes rocket, which is a peppery salad leaf. It has only recently regained the popularity it enjoyed in Ancient Rome. When seasoned with extra virgin olive oil, balsamic vinegar, pepper and finely chopped garlic, it is perhaps the most spritely salad available. It was recommended by the Roman poet Ovid, who called it salacious, and Martial, who wrote that it promoted amorous desire. It is now served in every fashionable restaurant and is readily available in supermarkets. It was dedicated to the god of sex and excess, Priapus, and sown around his statues. One Roman poet wrote:

'Hail, Priapus, near thee we sow
To rouse to duty husbands who are slow.'

Spinach has enjoyed a reputation on account of its rich iron content. Baby spinach is excellent as the basis

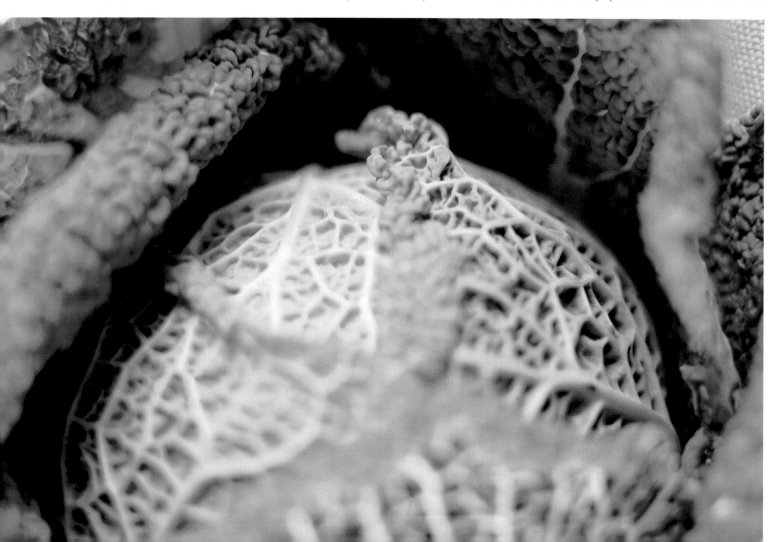

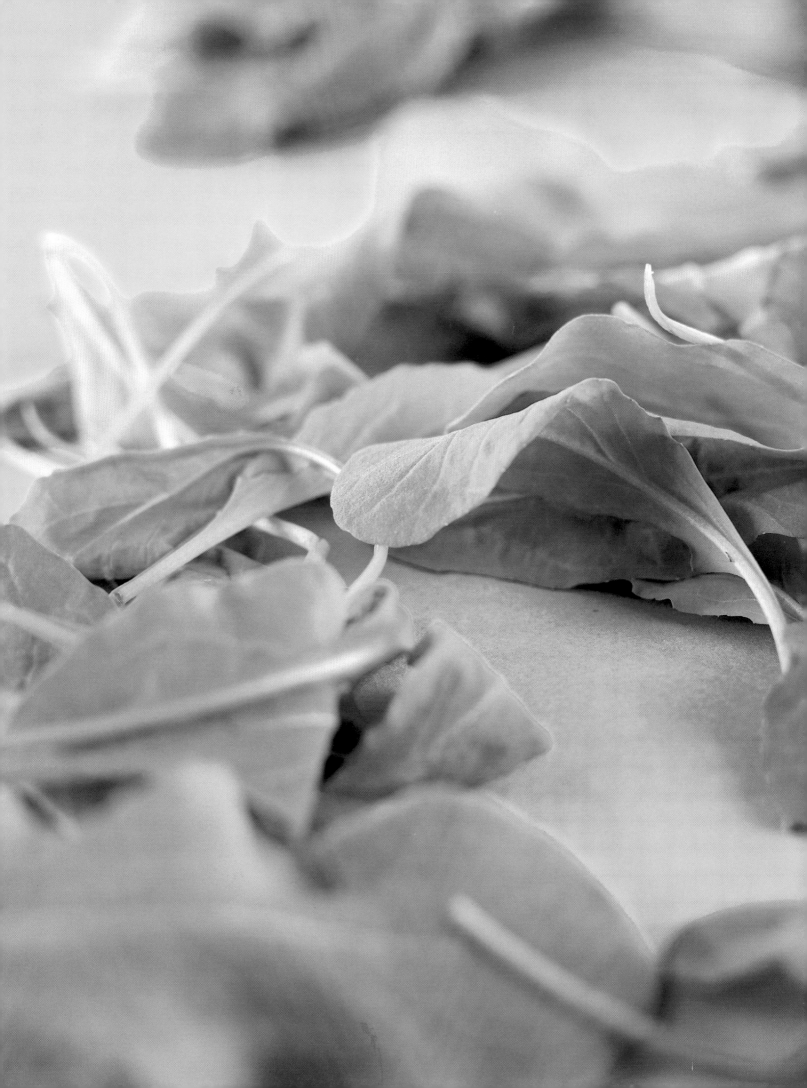

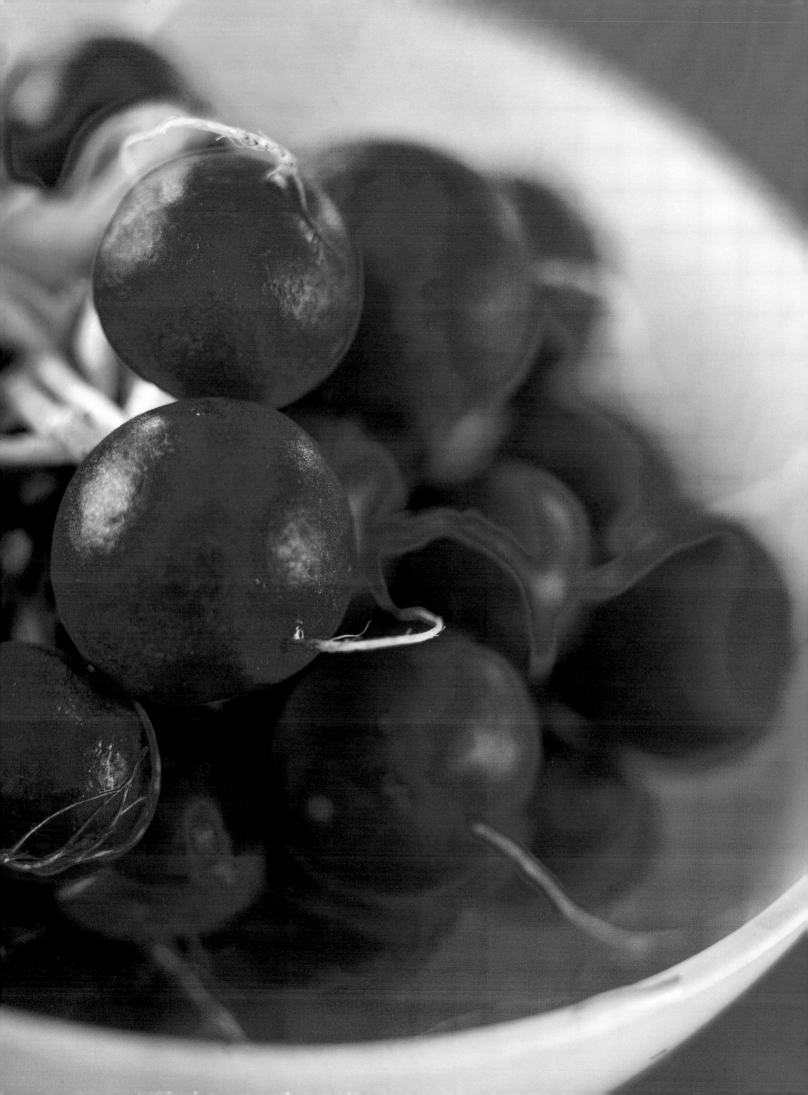

for a salad, especially if topped with croutons and crispy bacon. Cooking spinach should take no more than a few minutes, using only the water which sticks to the leaves after rinsing.

No salad is complete without some radishes to leave on the side of the plate. But historically they were held in high esteem as an aid to marital relations, so much so that Claude Bigothier published a poem in their honour, in 1540.

Salad vegetables

The Romans dedicated celery to Pluto, god of sex and the underworld. An unusual combination! In the Middle Ages it was used as a charm to produce male children. If it was placed under the bed of a pregnant woman without her knowledge and the first name she pronounced was that of a man, it guaranteed that the child would be a boy. Celery seeds concentrate the celery's aphrodisiac powers.

Crush them and add to a salad dressing, or best of all, sprinkle them on oysters to produce a lethal combination.

Celery soup was popular in the eighteenth century as a means of whetting the sexual appetite, for not only was it good for the blood, bursting with vitamins and minerals, but it also had rarity value. The cultivated version we now know has only been grown since the early years of the nineteenth century and its wild cousin was bitter and hardly palatable. For best advantage eat it raw, with dips such as houmous (see chick peas) or taramasalata (which features in the Seafood chapter), or in salads. It can also add zest to many soups such as Spring Vegetable, especially when you can use the young sprouting green leaves.

Watercress is the oddity of the salad bowl. Most salad vegetables are surprisingly anaphrodisiac. In his treatise on food in 1539, Sir Thomas Elyot wrote that 'Lettyse...increaseth mylke in a woman's breasts, but

OPPOSITE: RADISHES, DESPITE THEIR AFTER-EFFECTS, ARE HIGHLY REGARDED.

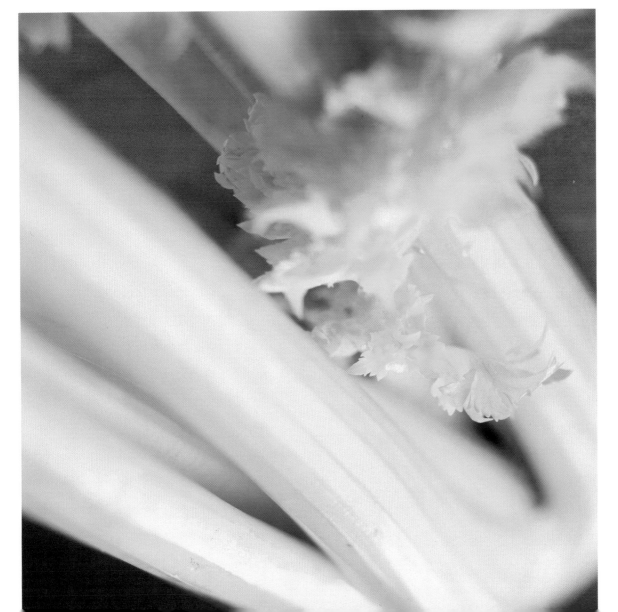

LEFT: CELERY, DEDICATED TO THE GOD OF SEX.

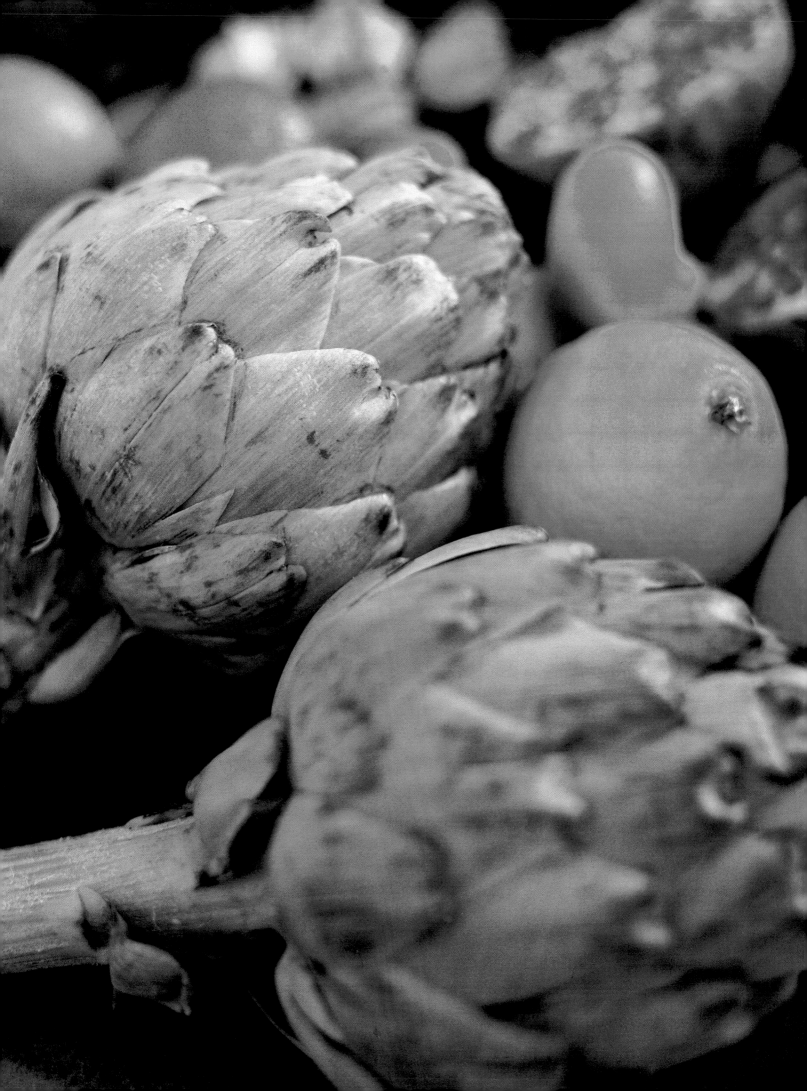

'Celery...our conscience obliges us to warn shy people to abstain from it, or at least use it prudently. It is enough to stress that it is not anyway a salad for bachelors'.
Grimod de la Reyière

abateth appetite.' But we know that salad vegetables can be part of a healthy diet. Watercress is a wonderful tonic and purifier of the blood and is one of the most versatile of garnishes. Combine it with a previously described aphrodisiac, the walnut, for heightened effect. Chop walnuts and mix them with a chopped apple, chopped spring onions (scallions) and some cheese of your choice. A smooth one, such as Gruyère or Gouda is best. Smother in a dressing of your choice. To make a more substantial lunch dish put in some chopped hard-boiled eggs and a few slivers of anchovy. Both add to the aphrodisiac qualities.

Other ideas

Globe artichokes were described by John Gerard in his *Herbal*, with meticulous advice on how to make the best of them: 'The middle pulp to be boiled with broth of fat flesh with added pepper to become a dainty dish being pleasant to the taste and accounted good to produce bodily desire. It stayeth the involuntary course of the natural seed'. The Law of Rarity applied to the globe artichoke, as in Gerard's time it was imported at considerable expense and was therefore only available at the tables of the rich and mighty. Now they are commonplace, but the ritual of eating them can be quite provocative.

Similarly, avocados were rare when first introduced into Europe from central America. Now very common, their high protein content, almost the highest in the vegetable kingdom, gives them restorative properties. You can eat them plain, serve with a good sprinkle of freshly ground black pepper, add a dressing of your choice, add a topping of prawns (another aphrodisiac) or make them into an unusual soup. Add the mashed flesh of two large ripe avocados to a pint of chicken stock. Heat and stir in cream to taste. Sieve to achieve a silky consistency, season with salt and pepper and sprinkle with ground mace.

They can be served with prawns or crab sitting atop a halved avocado, or use them to make an excellent salad base by mashing together with the seafood. Pop in some finely chopped celery and tarragon for texture. They can also be baked, but care must be taken not to reduce them to too soft a consistency. A little buffalo mozzarella cheese makes a suitable addition when cooked in this way.

Asparagus has long been thought of as a supreme aphrodisiac, both through the Doctrine of Signatures and the Law of Rarity, as previously defined. In the seventeenth century, the great herbalist, Culpeper, wrote that asparagus '...stirreth up bodily lust in man and woman'. Long before that, it makes an early appearance in *The Perfumed Garden*, in a rather

OPPOSITE: ARTICHOKES WERE ONCE A RARE APHRODISIAC, BUT ARE NOW COMMONPLACE.

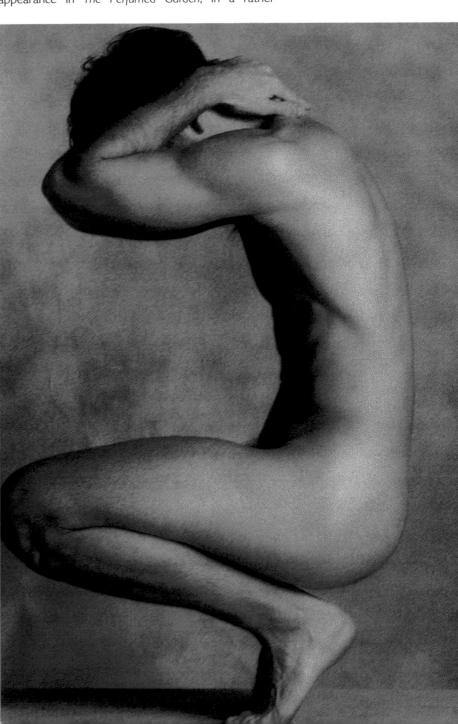

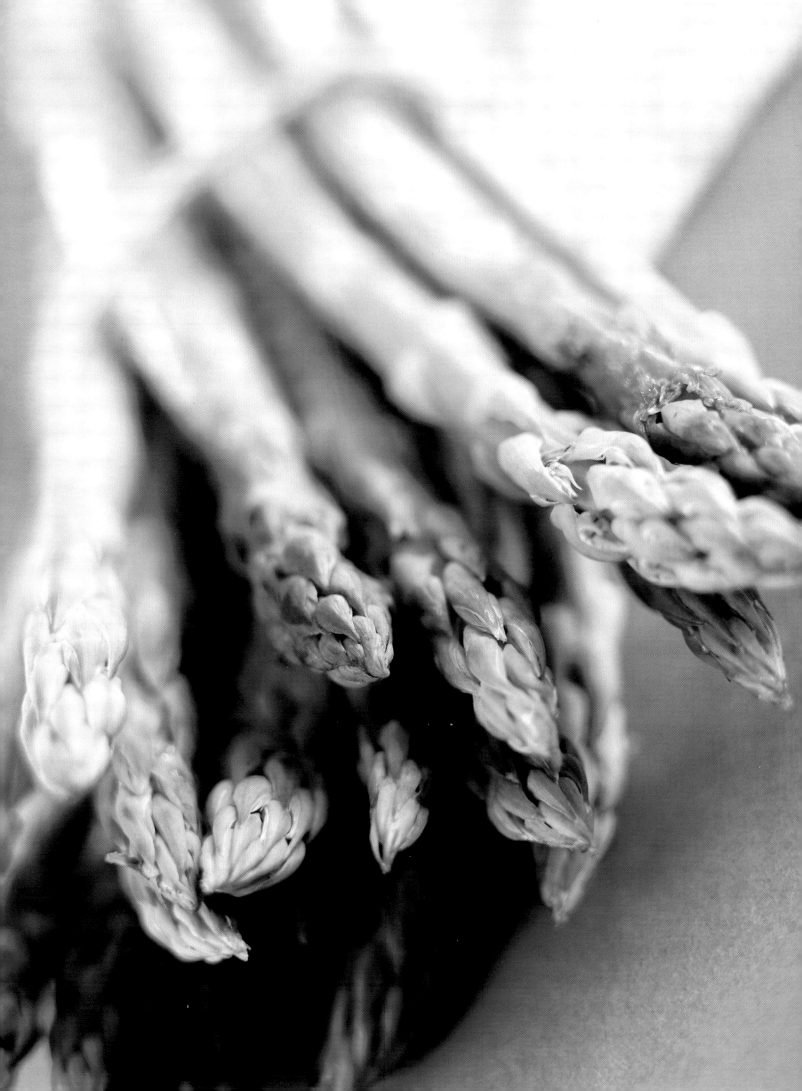

unpleasant form. Nefwazi suggested that it be boiled and then fried in fat with egg yolks and condiments – very cholesterol rich. It is best used fresh (few tinned foods are recommended for use as aphrodisiacs) and boiled, preferably in an asparagus boiler which allows the stem to be cooked tender without overcooking the tips. Alternatively, asparagus can be lightly grilled. Serve simply with lemon or melted butter. If a richer concoction is called for, mix two tablespoons of lemon juice with four egg yolks. Add a pinch of fresh, chopped tarragon, with seasoning to taste. A touch of cayenne gives it bite. Heat in a double boiler or in a bowl placed in a pan of hot water. Add about a quarter pound of butter in small pieces. Dribble over the freshly boiled asparagus. Eat with fingers, adding to the erotic effect.

A word of caution. The French aphrodisiac specialist Quensel warned, in 1809, that it can excite men, but can have the opposite effect on women.

As a base or side dish for these aphrodisiac dishes, rice is the perfect accompaniment. It has a long history as an aphrodisiac, the Hindu Ananga-Ranga suggested that a mixture of wild rice and honey should be eaten every evening. A more obscure recipe suggests boiling sparrow's eggs and rice in milk, to which honey and ghee (clarified butter) can be added. To update this dish, substitute with quail's eggs.

A Truffle Interlude

Let's drink to the health of truffle black;
In gratitude we must not lack.
For they assure us dominance
In all erotic dalliance.

17th Century French Eulogy

Truffles, alongside oysters, are often credited as one of the ultimate aphrodisiacs. They were well known to the Romans for their powerful effect, and Apicus records six ways of preparing them for optimum

OPPOSITE: ENTICING ASPARAGUS.

BELOW: TRUFFLE HUNTING IN FRANCE.

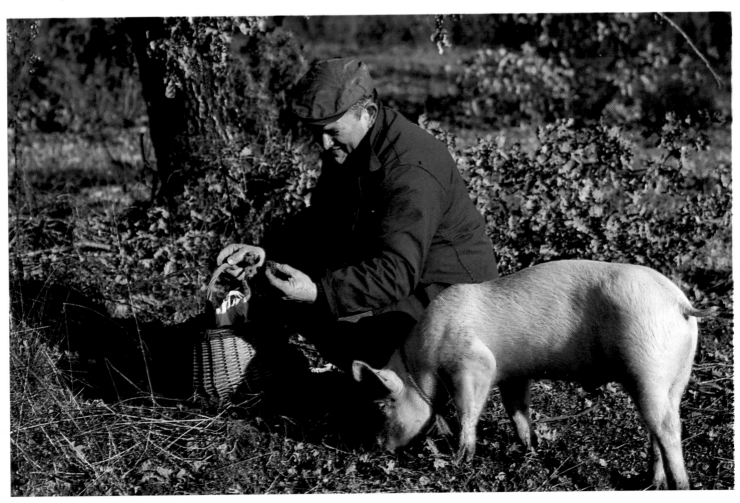

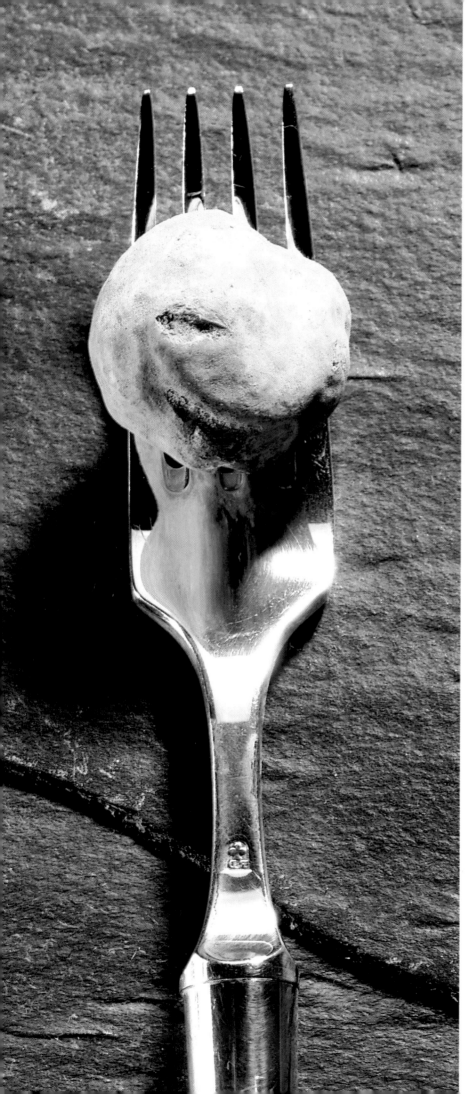

effect. Black truffles from France are the most prized, though many contend that the Italian white truffles, from Piedmont, are an even greater delicacy. The Romans preferred the highly-rated Libyan truffles. Pliny, fanciful as ever, speculated that they were so special that they must have been the result of a thunderbolt hitting the ground.

When the Roman Empire fell, the aphrodisiac properties of truffles were forgotten, or at least not recorded. The French revived interest in them in the eighteenth century and accorded them remarkable erotic powers. That most famous writer on food, Brillat-Savarin, devotes six pages in his classic work to the erotic tuber and provides an anecdote of how a lady narrowly escaped being ravished by a gentleman guest to whom she had served a hen stuffed with truffles.

Truffles have been favoured by the powerful, from Emperor Claudius to Madame de Pompadour. Louis XIV is recorded as having eaten a pound a day, whilst Napoleon's Marshals kept him virile with an ample supply.

The French writer, Colette, described truffles as the 'jewels of the poor soil'. Unearthed by pigs, who are drawn to the musky aroma, they are jewels indeed and command comparable prices. In the 1998 season the best fetched nearly £200 ($320) a pound in France. Perhaps they are the last example of the Law of Rarity, their exclusivity adding to their power. They are slowly becoming available in supermarkets – but even there, at a price.

Nothing much needs doing to a truffle other than to shave or chop it. A few flakes added to a simple dish of scrambled eggs transforms it into ambrosia. A heady combination of taste and aroma can provide a romantic aura, even before the magic of the truffle itself begins to work.

To reduce the expense, but still experience the truffle, find a bottle of good white truffle oil. Strongly infused with the truffle it will raise the spirits and the libido when drizzled over a favourite pasta or pizza.

LEFT: A FORTUNE'S WORTH OF TRUFFLE ON A SUITABLY GRAND FORK.

RIGHT: A SIMPLE WAY OF SERVING BABY ASPARAGUS SPEARS – WITH SCRAMBLED EGGS.

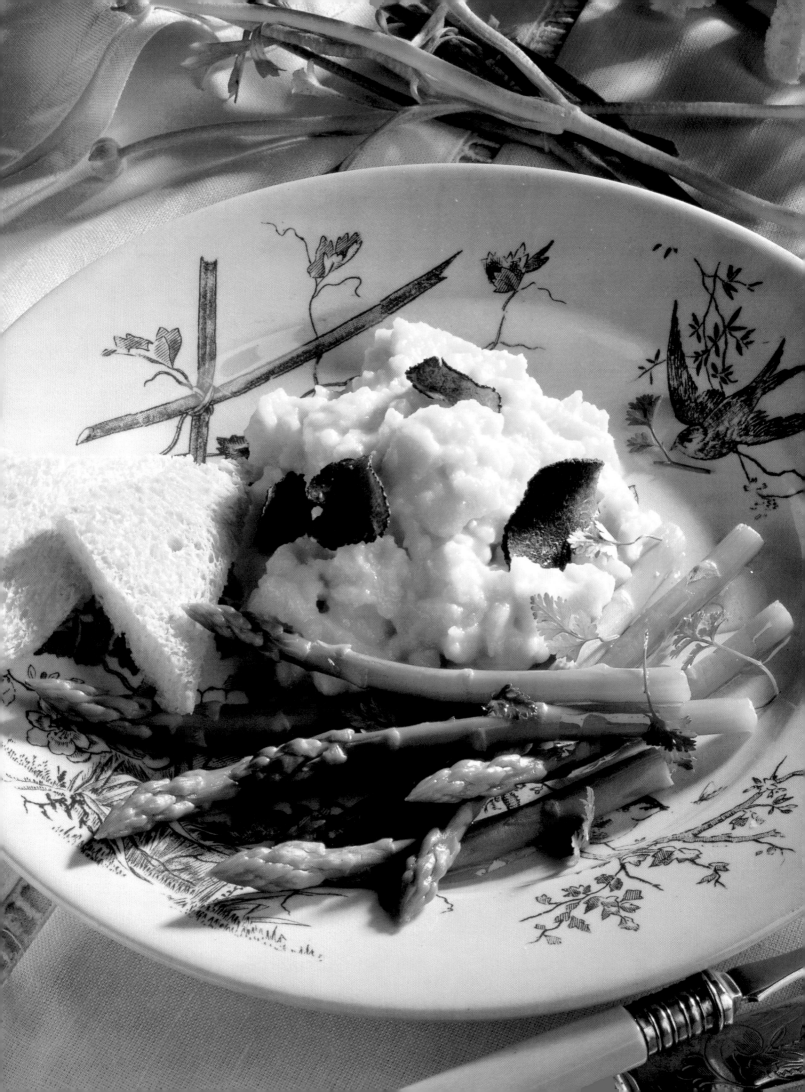

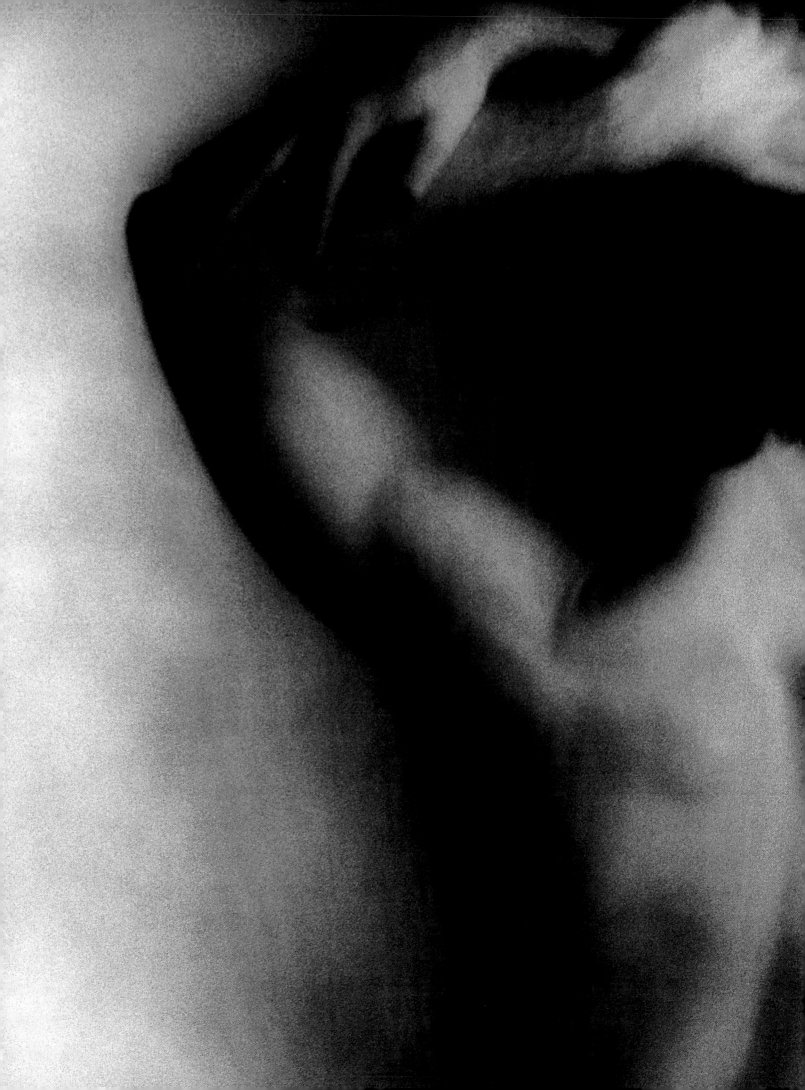

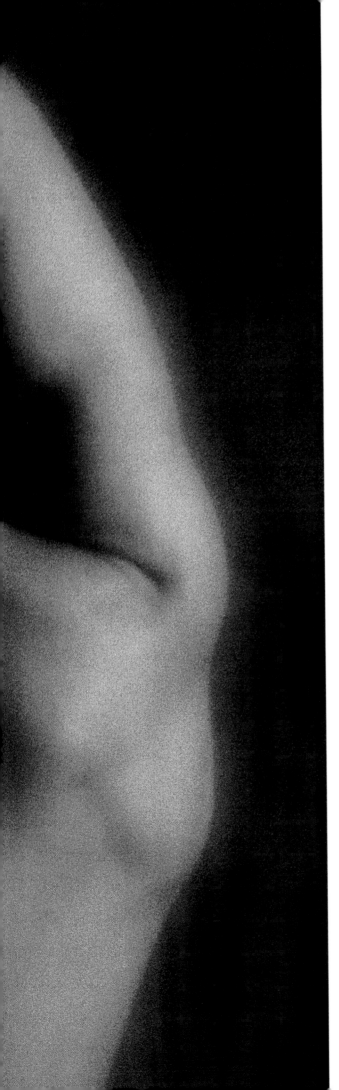

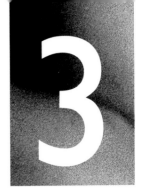

APHRODISIACS FROM SEA AND STREAM

When Aphrodite, the Greek goddess of Love, reputedly sprang from the sea on an oyster shell and promptly gave birth to Eros, the reputation of oysters as a powerful aphrodisiac was born. During the Roman Empire, their notoriety was such that Roman emperors paid for them by their weight in gold.

By the middle of the 17th century they were considered the very incarnation of aphrodisia. Casanova, it is said, was a firm believer in oysters, consuming fifty of them raw every morning in the bath, usually accompanied by the lady he had seduced the previous night. Presumably the oysters would reinvigorate him for the demands of the night to come.

Oysters

Is their reputation borne out by biological facts? Certainly oysters are low in fat and high in minerals and are therefore a particularly healthy food. They are also high in phosphorous, iodine and zinc, the latter being a noted promoter of testosterone production.

Oysters must have had a widespread effect as they were not subject to the Rule of Rarity until recent years. Indeed well into this century they were food for the masses. Charles Dickens had Sam Weller say that '…poverty and oysters always seem to go together.'

Even before consumption oysters look lascivious lying naked in their half-shell and the act of consumption heightens the effect. They are best taken *au naturel*, served simply with crushed ice and seaweed to heighten the salty tang of the sea. Fresh lemon juice or Worcestershire sauce are both admirable accompaniments. If a spicy sauce is favoured the best consists of finely chopped shallots softened in red wine vinegar. If you really like it hot, add a dash of chilli sauce. An unusual way of enjoying your oyster is to take a fresh oyster, put it in a schnapps glass (a miniature tumbler), add a dash of fresh grated horseradish and a drop of chilli sauce. Top up with a shot of vodka, and knock back in one go to feel an almost immediate benefit.

Oysters can of course be baked or deep-fried in the Chinese fashion. It is generally thought that these methods destroy the aphrodisiac chemicals and the oysters are certainly not so suggestive to eat.

OPPOSITE: OYSTERS
AU NATUREL.

BELOW: BOTTICELLI'S
THE BIRTH OF VENUS.

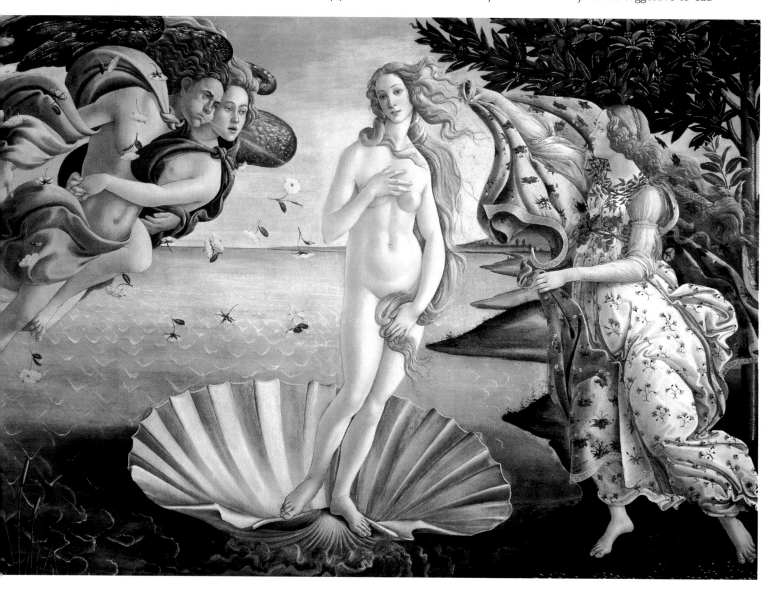

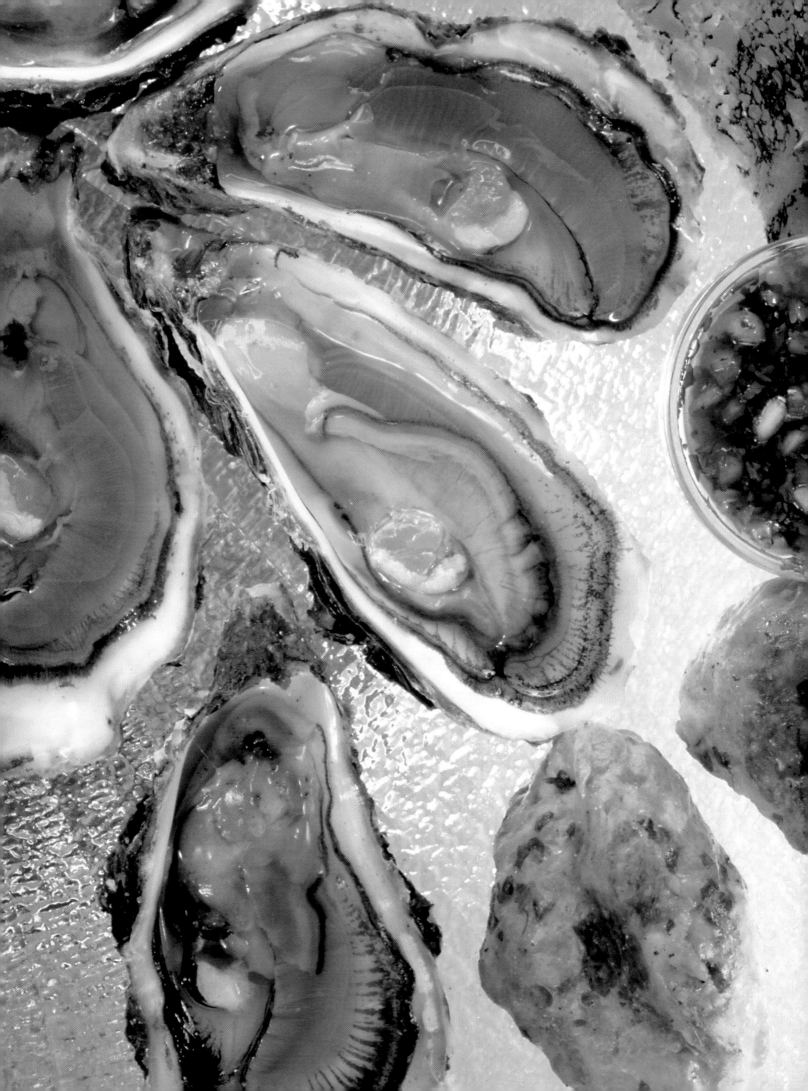

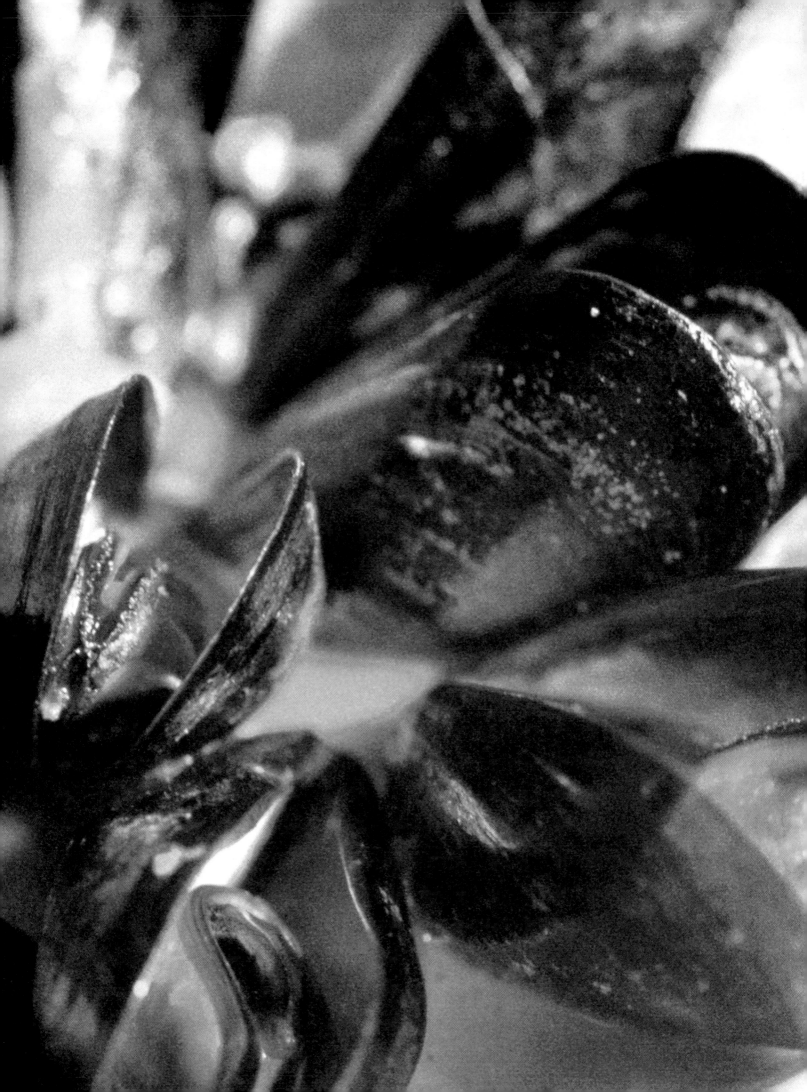

If the tang of the sea is not to your taste look out for freshwater oysters from Ireland or Australia. Nowhere do they taste sweeter than at the Rock Pool restaurant near Sydney harbour.

Other seafoods

Other beneficial seafoods include cockles and clams, indeed almost everything which you would find in a sumptuous seafood platter, never more seductive than when eaten at La Timonerie, aon Cap d'Antibes, overlooking the azure Mediterranean. In general you can't go wrong with seafood.

Mussels are, for reasons lost in the mists of time, associated with Belgium. But for aphrodisiac effects one must look further south to Italy where they are known as cozza, a name with intimate female connotations.

They can be eaten raw, just like oysters, but produce best results when joined with garlic and butter in a rich cooked sauce. Pickling them in brine negates any positive effect they may have. The kings of the mussel world are the large green-shelled mussels of New Zealand, best eaten at the restaurant Cin-Cin on Auckland harbour

Anchovies, both fresh or preserved in brine or oil, are one of the most versatile of fishes. Their salty tang adds something lascivious to many dishes. Like so many aphrodisiacs they have been recognised as such since Roman times. In Britain, the Victorians were particularly partial to them. And we know what carnal lusts lurked in their breasts.

A portmanteau meal, combining many aphrodisiacs, bound together with anchovies, is the Venus Sandwich.

OPPOSITE: WITHIN THE SHELLS OF MOLLUSCS LIE THE STUFF OF APHRODISIA.

BELOW: CAVIAR – BLACK GOLD FROM THE VIRGIN STURGEON.

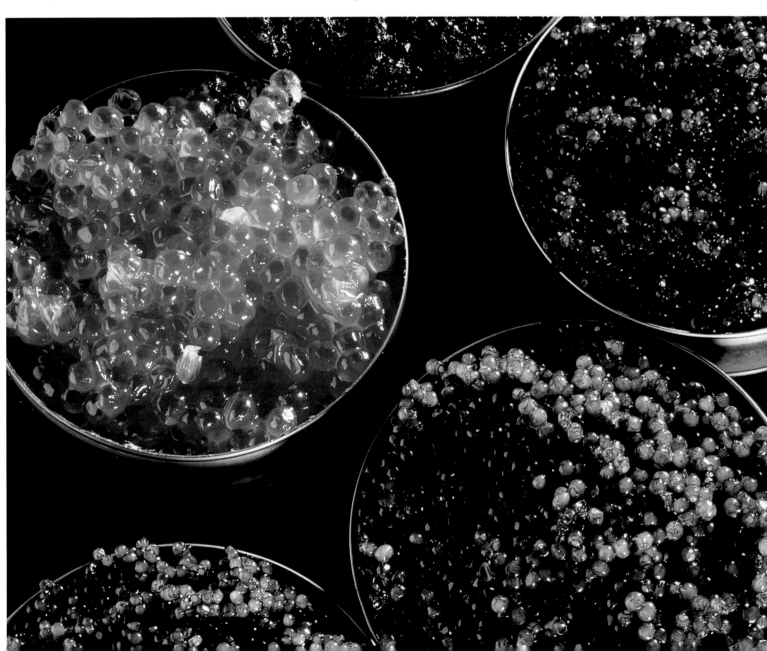

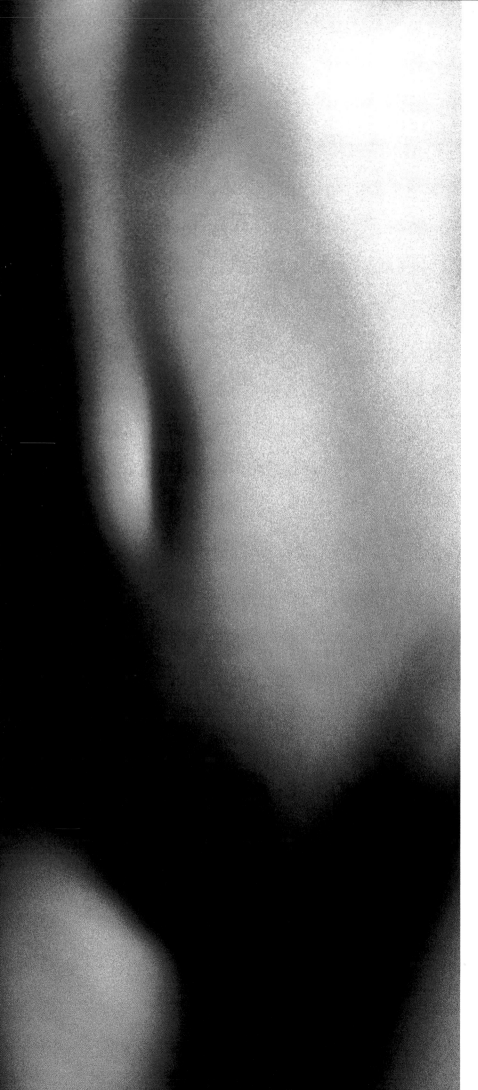

Take a French loaf, slice part way through. Scoop out some of the white bread. Drizzle well with good olive oil. Then fill it with a mountain of anchovies (tinned ones work well), stoned black olives, capers, roughly chopped, skinned and de-seeded tomatoes and whatever else takes your fancy. Artichoke hearts or asparagus tips add a touch of class. Leave it to marinate under a weight for an hour or so. The juices will mingle and infuse the bread. Eat messily, with a companion of your choice. Juices dribbling down the chin as you eat always adds to the aphrodisiac effect.

If you take your anchovies relatively straight try Anchovy Toasts. Fry some fingers of bread, then lay an anchovy fillet on each. Sprinkle, or flake, some parmesan on top. Put in a hot oven for a few minutes.

With a reputation second only to the noble oyster comes caviar; Beluga, Sevruga or Osietra. Sturgeon roe has remained the food of kings and certainly obeys the Rule of Rarity. There is precious little to do with caviar other than eat it straight. Serve in a silver dish on a bed of ice. Use a small silver spoon to eat it straight. Allow the eye to enjoy the sight of the small, black shiny eggs, before alternating tiny spoonfuls with sips of champagne or ice-cold vodka. If a garnish is considered necessary have a little chopped hard-boiled egg yolk and finely chopped onion on the side, to enhance the aphrodisiac effect. If you want to go for gold, one of Canada's most famous seafood bars suggests serving a blob of caviar atop each oyster. Gilding the lily?

There are other roes to hoe, lumpfish especially. It appears on every buffet. There is no reason to suppose that they do not have the same potency as caviar, as they are basically the same thing. But then the fish from whence they came was not the mighty sturgeon, surging through the icy waters of the Caspian sea.

The most popular dish based on roe is Taramasalata. It is basically cod roe mixed to a smooth paste with olive oil, lemon juice and black pepper. Cream cheese can also be included, as well as a dash of paprika for colour.

RIGHT: BARBECUED PRAWNS BECOME SEXIER AS THEY CHANGE HUE FROM GREY TO LUSCIOUS PINK.

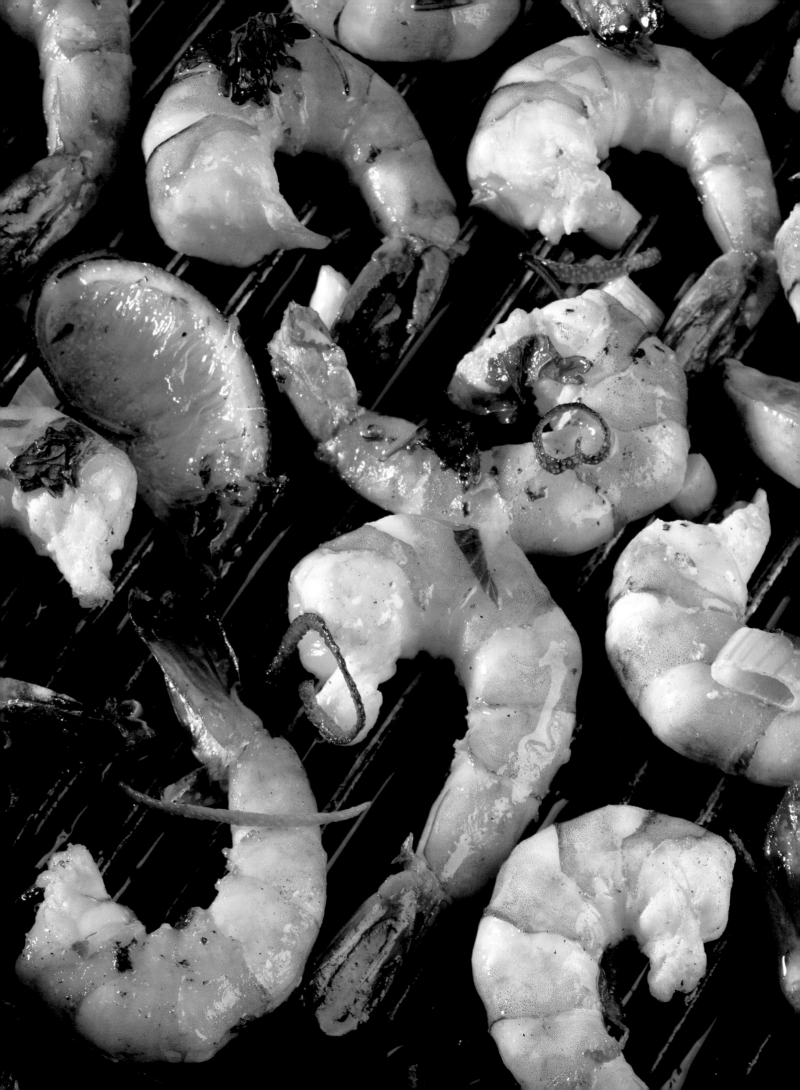

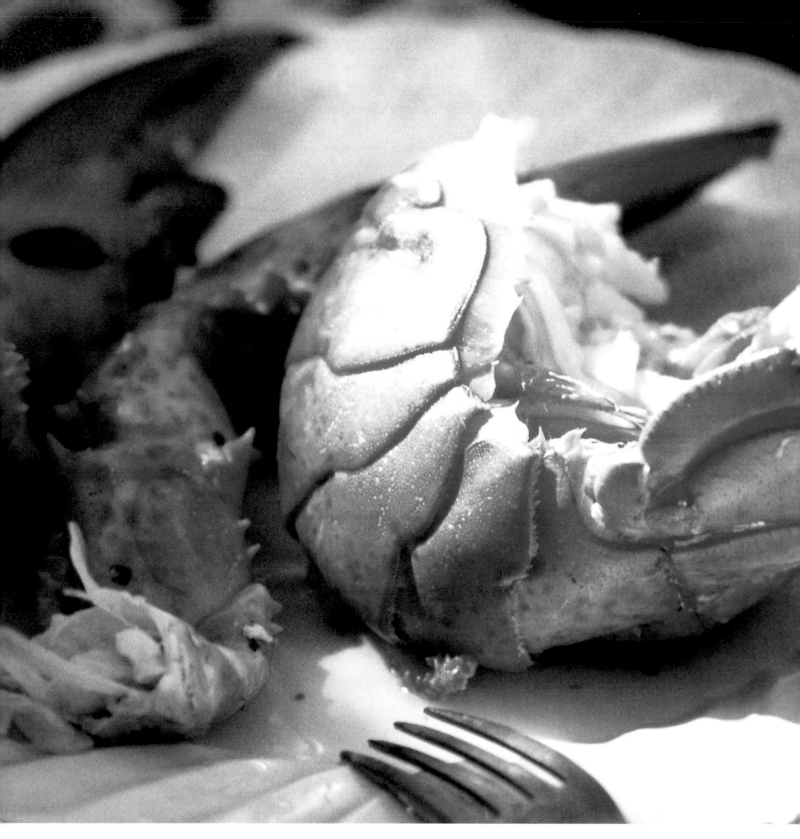

Shrimps and prawns

From the tiniest shrimp to the mighty oyster, the oceans play a large part in the world of aphrodisia. Don't baulk at the thought of the ubiquitous prawn cocktail. Rubbery prawns in a violent pink sauce do nothing for anyone's love life, so re-invent the dish with plump tiger prawns, smothered in a smooth sauce made of home-made mayonnaise coloured only with a dash of paprika and a squeeze of lemon, served on a bed of the crispiest lettuce.

We are used to buying our shrimps ready cooked, but for barbecues, or eating al fresco, raw ones are best, even if frozen. Watching them change from dirty grey to dusky pink as they cook is strangely alluring. From New Zealand comes Shrimp Piri Piri. Peel and vein the raw prawns. Cook briefly in a little white wine with herbs of your choice. Try bay leaf and perhaps a dash of lemon for zest. Serve on sticks, with a dip, which can range from Guacamole (the powerful mashed avocado, with a dash of chilli), to a concentrated tomato relish with peppers.

Lobster and crab

Lobster may make for hard work. For a suggestive meal be prepared to demolish the creature at table. One ready prepared from a supermarket may provide the essential nutrients, but does not create the much-needed ambience. Tearing flesh from claws, poking around its inner bits, or cracking claws with various implements, creates a positively hot-house atmosphere.

There are classic cooked lobster dishes, particularly those enhanced with lashings of brandy. A sensual treat is Lobster Shepherd's Pie created at the Union Square Café in New York. Chunks of lobster meat are layered between mashed potato and carrot, those vegetable aphrodisiacs. But nothing beats the creature unadorned.

Crabs require similar violent and suggestive treatment at table. Standard dressed crab is not erotic to eat, though both brown and white meats are said to encourage passion. Follow the style of London's Caprice restaurant. In a round mould, shape the white meat with a decent mayonnaise, seasoned with a dash of mace. Layer in a little chopped hard-boiled egg yolk.

CRACK A CLAW FOR CARNALITY.

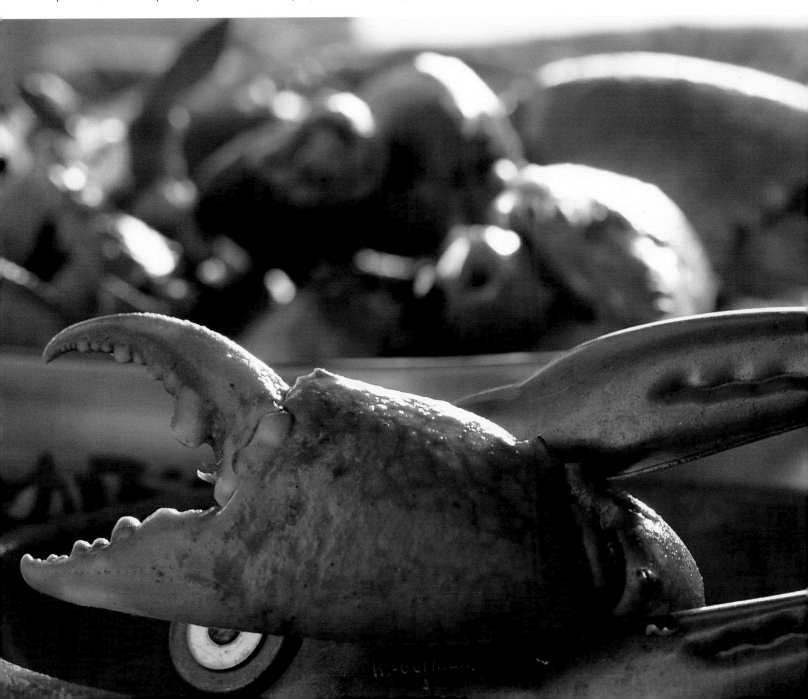

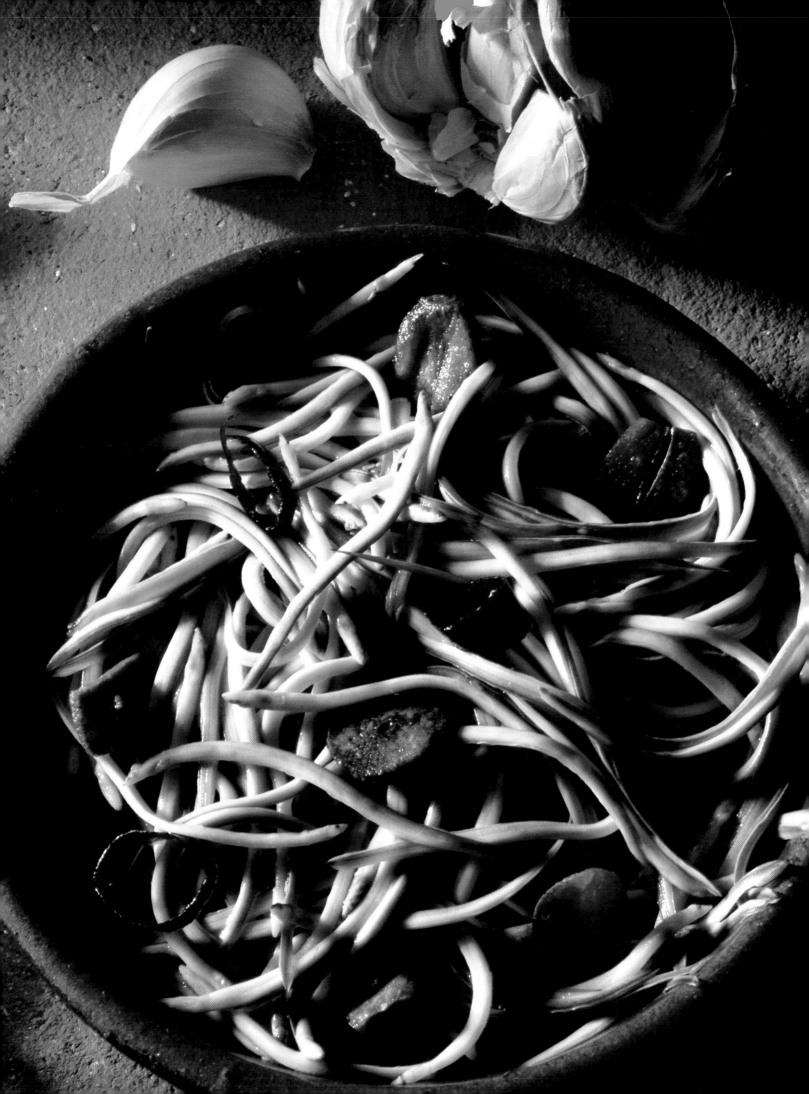

Top with a layer of brown meat laced with a dash of good brandy. Remove the mould and you have a glorious mountain of concentrated richness.

Eels

Eels are not to everyone's taste, even though they blatantly proclaim the Doctrine of Similarities. Eel is a firm, chewy flesh, especially when smoked. If you are a little squeamish try a simple eel soup. Simmer bite-sized, cleaned eel for 20 minutes in ample water with some salt, a few peppercorns and a bay leaf. Make a roux of flour and butter (put simply, that means melt the butter and then cook the flour in it). Add the water in which the eel has cooked and simmer for a further 15 minutes. Return the eel to the liquid and throw in some roughly chopped parsley. Reheat gently. If you don't mind the high cholesterol, beat in two egg yolks before serving.

Another dish which gives you the goodness of eel without having anything too eel-like on your plate, is Italian Eel Bake. Again trim and cut your eel into bite size pieces. Sauté some finely sliced onions and red peppers in sufficient vegetable oil in an oven-proof casserole. Add the eel pieces, a glass of dry white wine, the juice of a lemon and seasoning. Bake in a hot oven for about 10 minutes. Then add some butter and a good sprinkling of parmesan or some similar hard cheese, peccarino for example. Bake for a further five minutes. Garnish with more fresh parsley and serve with polenta or potato – anything that will absorb the glorious juices.

Other ideas

Scandinavians sustain their erotic prowess with the help of the humble herring. The number of ways they pickle them are seemingly countless. Witness the dozens of barrels of them which entice you on the quaysides of Copenhagen, Stockholm or Oslo. Their aphrodisiac secret lies in their oiliness, a virtue they share with the equally humble mackerel. Filleted and grilled these two fish may not seem that romantic, but they provide plenty of tastebud stimulation.

Octopus, squid and their various relations are aphrodisiacs, particularly when cooked in their own black ink. The ink itself can also be used to make a visually arresting and exotic risotto or black pasta in Italy. Cook gently or you will end up with an unappealing grey dish that will do nothing for your sex life.

Many countries and regions have made use of a variety of seaweeds to use as aphrodisiacs. In Wales, seaweed is served as laver bread. In Japan it is dried and served as a side-dish to raw fish sushi and sashimi dishes. In Chinese cuisine abalone is rated highly, but it is definitely an acquired taste. It lives within a shell, which sticks to rocks rather like a limpet sticks to ships. It needs gentle preparation unless you want the offputting experience of eating something akin to a chunk of rubber tyre.

The Japanese know the value of raw fish as aphrodisiacs. They are recorded in their sex manuals, the *Pillow Books*, and enjoy huge popularity today. Taken plain and sliced, sashimi includes well-known fish such as tuna, salmon and halibut, alongside more exotic creations. Sea urchin is highly prized, but not, as yet, a firm favourite in the West. Sushi involves serving the raw fish on a roll of moist rice, with seaweed on the side. A trio of aphrodisiacs.

Eating fish raw enhances its aphrodisiac properties. Technically speaking céviche and other marinated fish dishes are 'cooked'. The effect of the marinade, drizzled over the fine slices of fish, is to cook them, as is evidenced by the change of colour and texture. Céviche, strictly speaking, should be made with finely sliced cod, but popular variations involve salmon and tuna or sliced king scallops.

To help slice the fish finely, place it in a freezer for a short time to firm it up. Do not allow it to freeze. Make a marinade of extra virgin olive oil, balsamic

OPPOSITE AND BELOW: JAPANESE SUSHI AND SASHIMI DEPLOY FRESH SEAFOOD FOR AN APHRODISIACAL EFFECT.

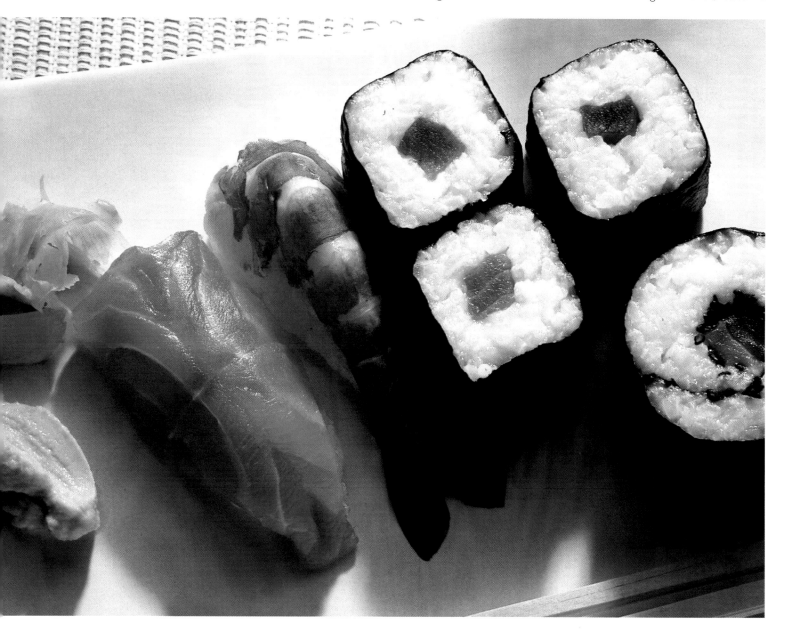

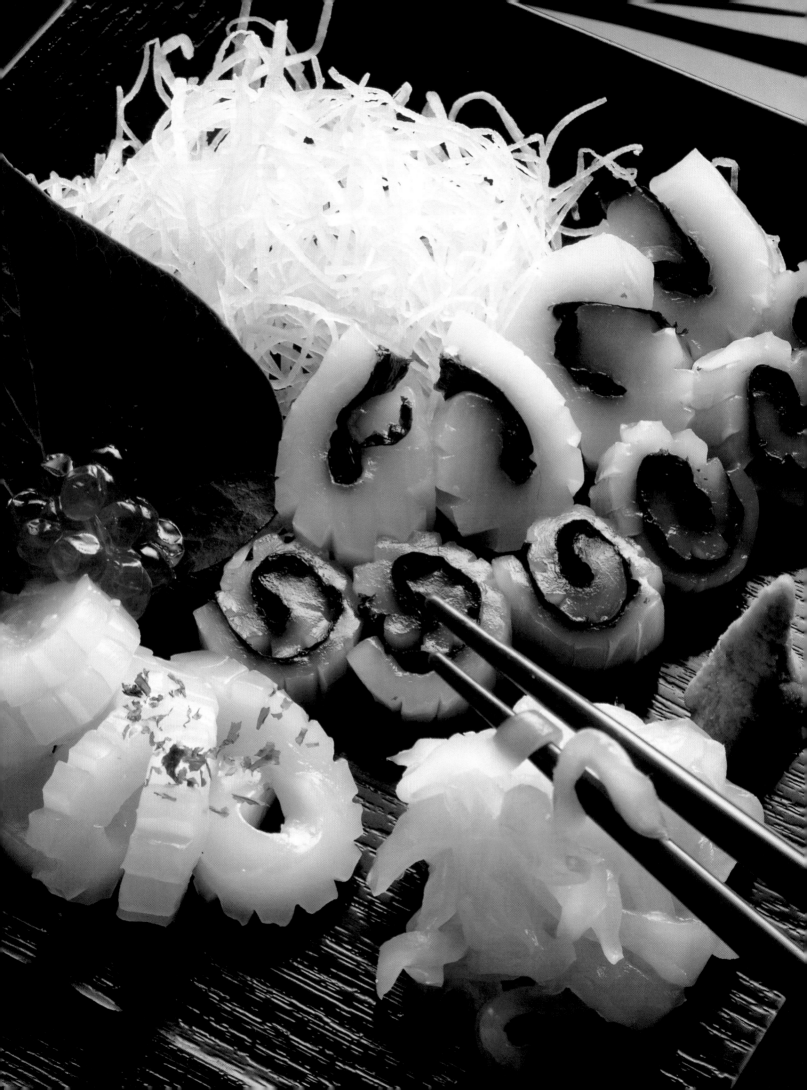

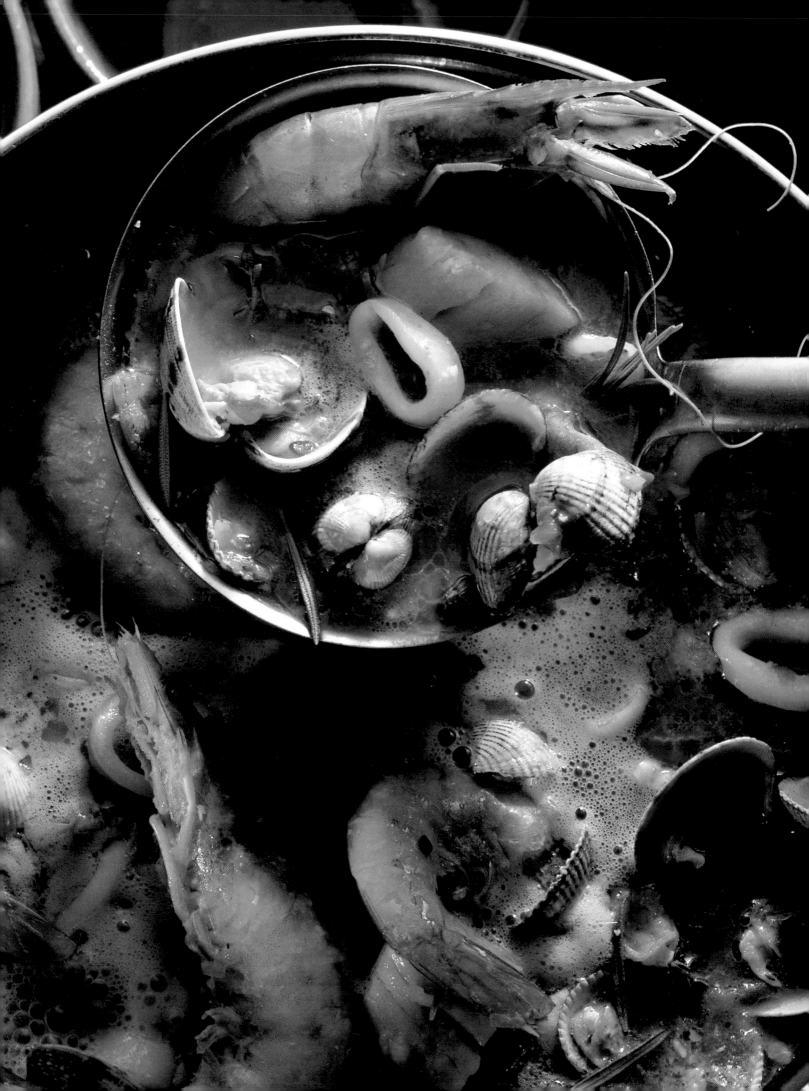

vinegar, some pink peppercorns and any other herb or spice you think will enhance a suitably amorous occasion. Dill is good with salmon and chilli can bring out the meatiness of tuna. Leave to marinade in a refrigerator for a couple of hours. The silkiness of marinaded fish is definitely sensual.

Fish stews

There is one dish that gives you full licence to plunder the aphrodisiac properties of the oceans. This is fish stew in its many forms. The Provençale dish, bouillabaisse, gives greatest scope for improvisation. In a large pan fry some onions, chopped leeks, garlic and tomatoes in olive oil until all are seductively golden. Then add a sprig of fennel, a sprig of thyme and some grated orange peel. Cook for another five minutes. Bring four pints (2.3 litres) of water to the boil, really bubbling, and add to the oil and vegetables. Whisk until it thickens. A dash more olive oil might add to the consistency. Now start adding your fish selection. Oily fish such as mackerel fillets or turbot go in first, followed by any shell fish you like, soft-shell crabs, prawns, clams etc. Soft white fish goes in last as they require only a few minutes to cook. Then add the supreme ingredient, a few strands, or a sachet, of saffron to give the dish a wonderful colour and intense aroma. Strain the fish from the liquid, retaining sufficient to keep it moist. Start your meal with the soup, served garnished with rouille (a garlic and chilli paste) and aioli (a garlic, egg yolk and olive oil mixture akin to mayonnaise), all extra-aphrodisiac. Follow by serving your mixed fish with plain boiled potatoes. Of course, mopping up the liquid with some garlic bread only adds to the experience.

OPPOSITE: A SEAFOOD STEW IS APHRODISIACAL HEAVEN.

BELOW: A SCENE FROM KITAGAWA UTAMARO'S *POEM OF THE PILLOW*.

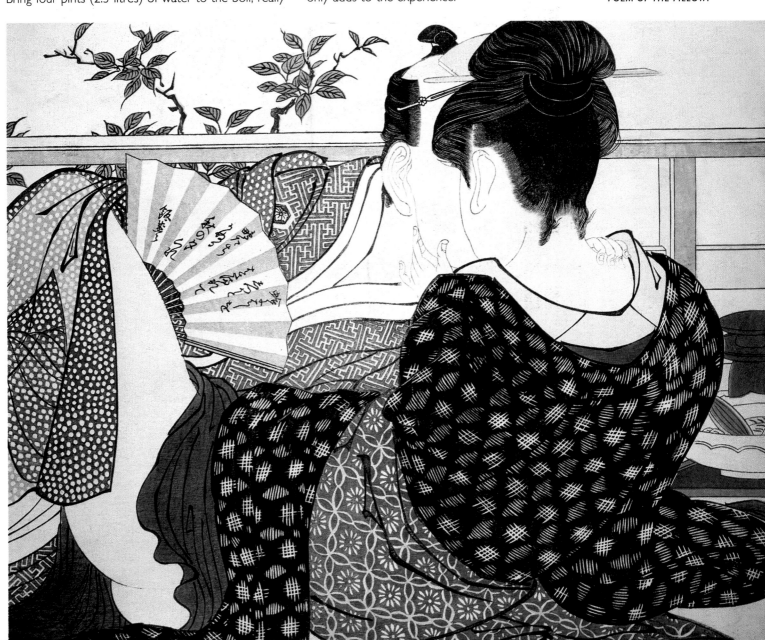

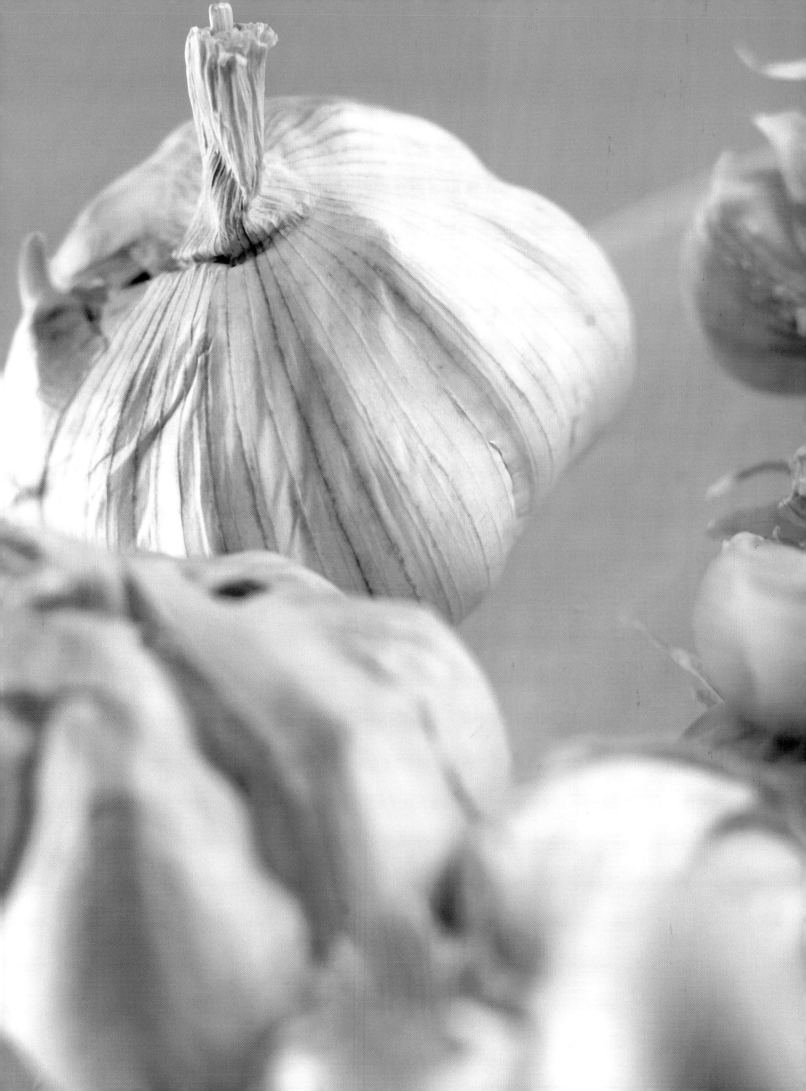

A Pungent Interlude

Already garlic has featured heavily in previous recipes, as befits its powerful aphrodisiac nature. Garlic evokes the warm Mediterranean and the passionate people of the countries which border it. But it is also found in the Orient, and indeed its wild form is a pestilent weed in many countries. It is the bulbous root of the genus Allium and has been worshipped as one of the holy trinity of aphrodisiacs alongside the truffle and the oyster. The Ainu people of Japan revere it in the same way as the Greeks revered nectar and ambrosia. Food of the gods.

In medieval England it was used not only to flavour poor quality food, but was thought to ward off the plague and relieve the symptoms if you caught it. Its many virtues include purifying the blood, cleaning the internal organs and building up strength and stamina. All of these virtues must contribute to its reputation as a major player in the aphrodisiac world.

It is the oil contained in this root that is the active ingredient, when it is taken for medicinal or aphrodisiac reasons. Its pungent smell can be repugnant to some, but it is positively addictive to many. If the smell really does upset, garlic pills are available, but they rather detract from the whole purpose of the exercise.

Garlic can be used in many ways. It enhances so many dishes, but can be particularly effective with young spring lamb roasts. Simply roasting the unpeeled bulb itself produces succulent cloves, which can be preserved in good olive oil for use in salads.

The ultimate garlic dish is Chicken with Fifty Cloves of Garlic. Take one free-range chicken and put some bay leaves, thyme sprigs and parsley inside it. Place some rosemary, chopped sage, and a couple of celery stalks into a deep pot. For added flavour you can include the giblets if you like them. Take fifty cloves of fresh garlic and place them at the bottom of the pot. Pour over some good olive oil and season. Put the chicken on top. Use a pot with a tight-fitting lid and seal as best as possible. Cook in a low oven for one and a half hours. Test the chicken by piercing between leg and breast. When the juices run clear it is ready. When done, arrange on a platter surrounded by the garlic. Serve with a crisp green vegetable, such as French beans or broccoli and big baked croutons. Take some slices of good plain white bread, brush with olive oil and perhaps a little pesto (the Italian basil, pine nut and olive oil paste) and place in a moderate oven until golden. Carve the chicken and place on the crouton to absorb the juices.

The power of the garlic is greatly enhanced by the herbs, most of which have aphrodisiac qualities of their own.

OPPOSITE: GARLIC HAS BEEN USED IN A HOST OF APHRODISIACAL DISHES SINCE ANCIENT TIMES.

BELOW: GARLIC WITH CHICKEN – AN EROTIC COMBINATION.

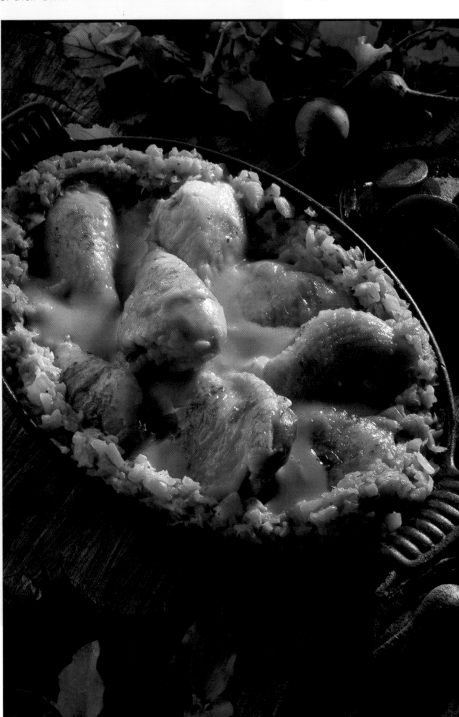

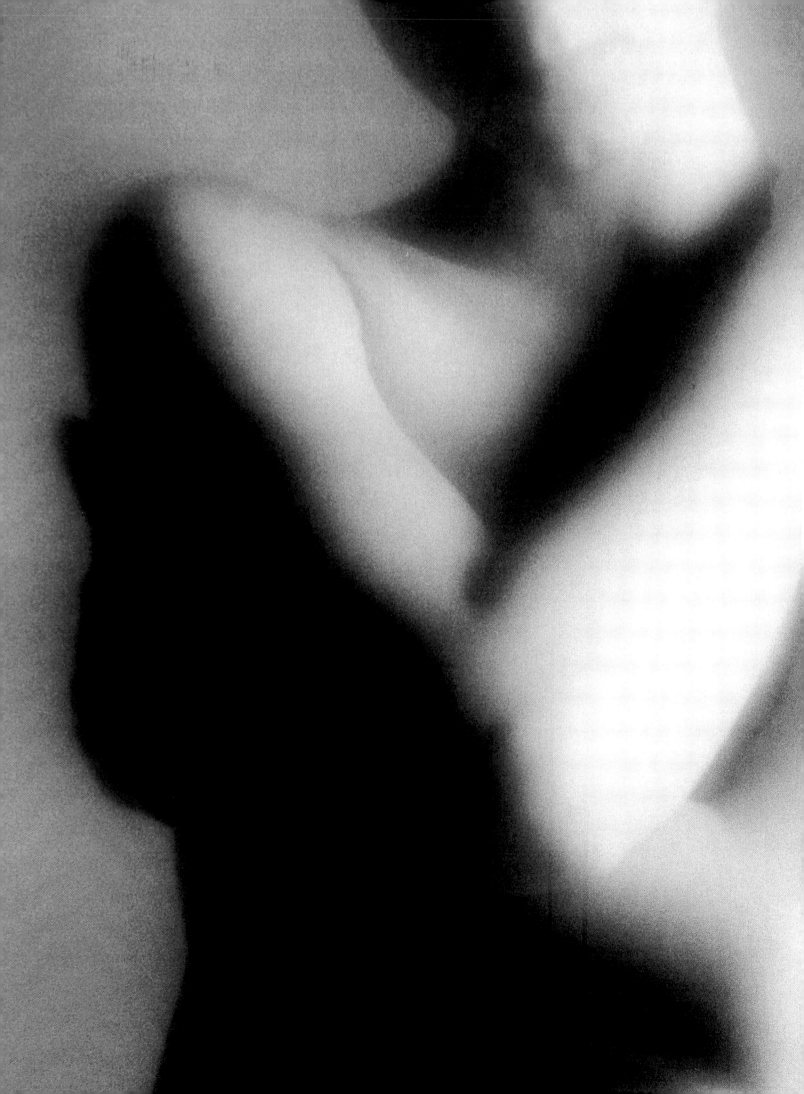

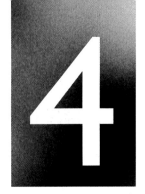

MEAT AND GAME APHRODISIACS

The Ancients laid great store in the aphrodisiac powers of meat in all shapes and forms. They particularly prized offal, especially the sexual organs of animals. Even today, cultures such as the Chinese still use some of these ingredients in recipes and medicines to promote increased sexual drive. However, even if they are effective, there is not much point in elaborating on such dishes here! Suffice it to say that there are many more palatable options available, which we will now explore.

Beef

Beef is a mighty aphrodisiac. The sheer sight of a whole Baron of Beef, on the bone of course, creates an atmosphere of lust, as well as providing the necessary calories for sustained performance. Do not over-indulge as a couple of good, bloody slices should suffice. To add to the allure, coat with a mixture of honey and whole grain mustard when roasting. A simple unadorned grilled slice of fillet is recommended, or even better is the classic dish, Beef Wellington. Though extremely glamorous, it is incredibly simple to prepare. Take a substantial piece of well-hung fillet. Trim off all sinews and fat (there should be little, anyway). Roll out some bought puff pastry (life is too short to make it – you could even buy ready-rolled). Seal the fillet quickly in a little, very hot, oil. Allow to cool. Place in the centre of the pastry. Put as generous a coating of pâté de foie gras, or any liver pâté, if times are hard, as you can on top of the fillet. Make a parcel of the pastry around it. Brush with beaten egg or milk. Bake in a medium oven until the pastry is golden brown. By this time the pâté will have moistened and coated the beef, which should be of pleasing rareness.

OPPOSITE: *AN ALLEGORY OF THE SENSE OF TASTE,* **BY JAN BRUEGHEL THE ELDER.**

BELOW: BEEF WELLINGTON COMBINES SUCCULENT FILLET OF BEEF WITH RICH PÂTÉ DE FOIE GRAS.

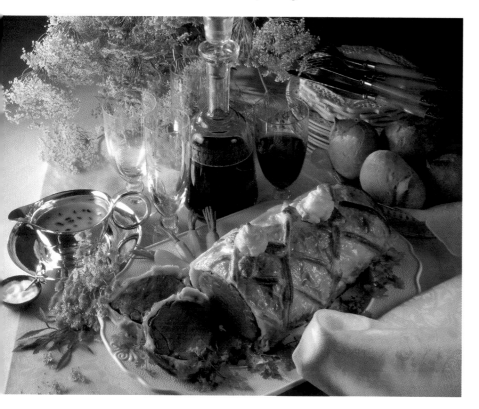

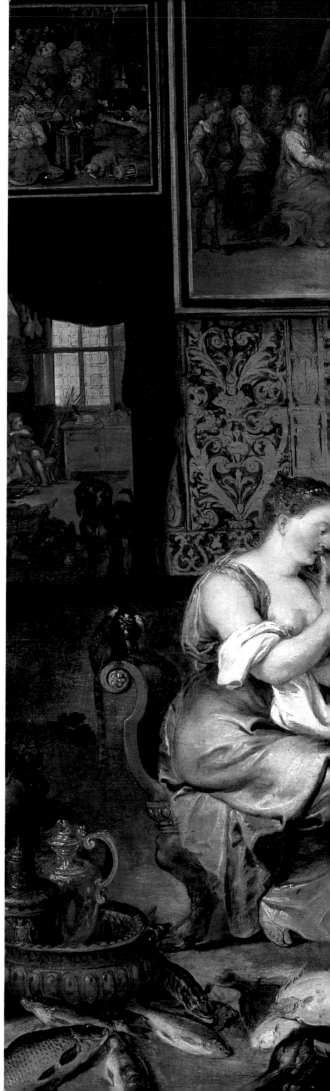

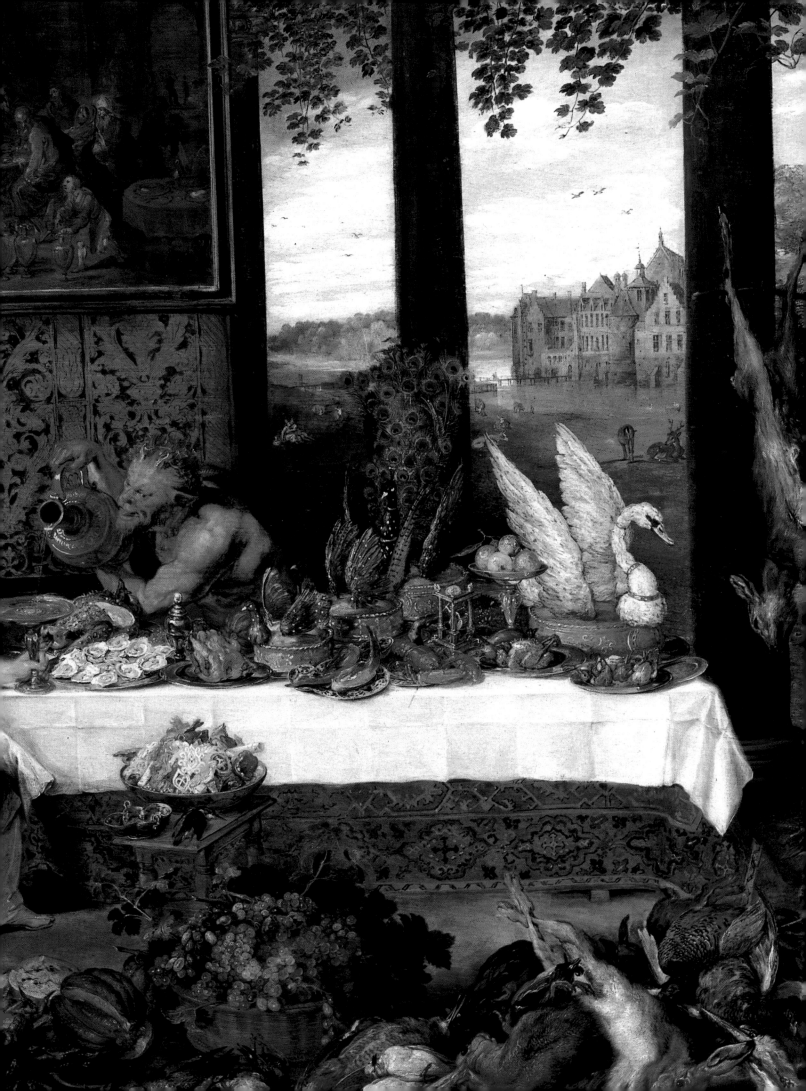

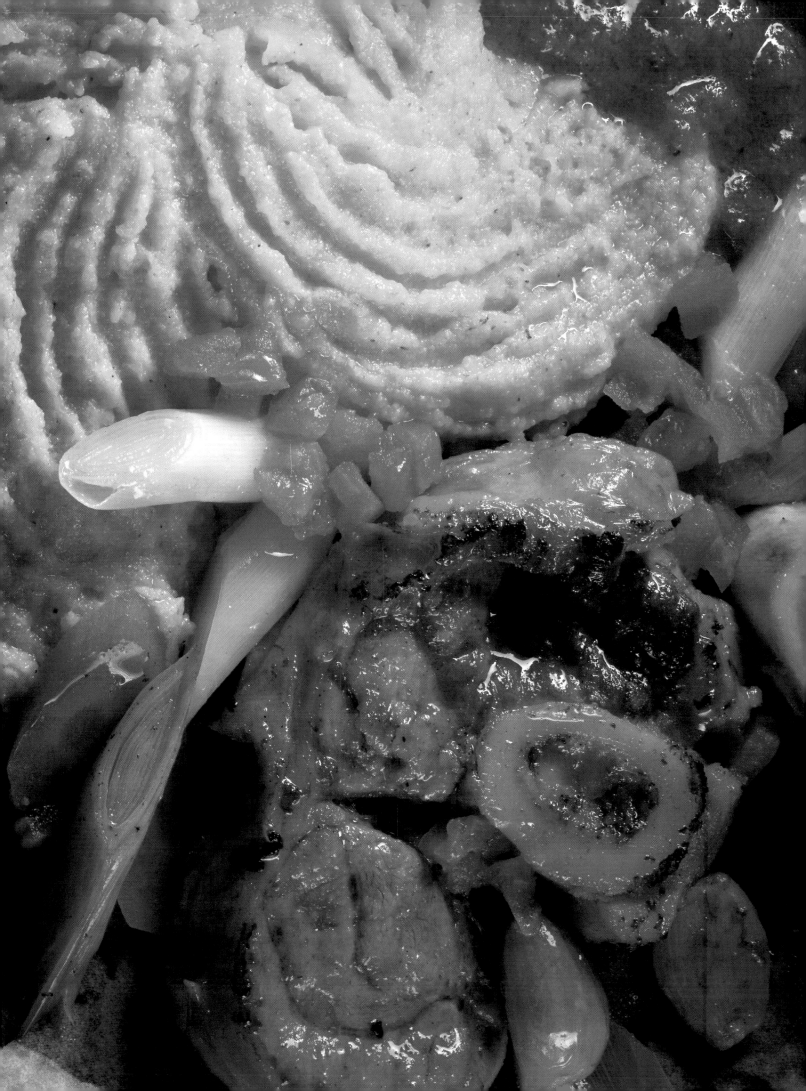

The best way of maximising the effect of fillet is to eat it raw, carpaccio in the Italian style. Buy a superb piece of fillet. Make a marinade of extra virgin olive oil, balsamic vinegar, a dash of wine vinegar, some peppercorns or coarse ground pepper. Bathe the fillet in this for a couple of hours, turning regularly to ensure that the outer layer of the fillet 'cooks'. Chill further in the freezer until it is firm enough to slice finely. Do not allow to freeze. Serve the slices with a tiny new potato and rocket salad.

Other variations

The other raw beef dish is Steak Tartare. Its antecedents are offputting, but today's version is extremely aphrodisiac. The nomadic races united under Attila the Hun put the raw beef between the saddle and their horse. By mealtime, which often took place after as long as a day's ride, it had been reduced to a bloody, but edible, mess. Don't let this thought put you off enjoying finely minced fillet steak, served with a raw egg yolk and some finely chopped onion for you to lasciviously mush up yourself. Don't let the waiter do it for you. It dampens the aphrodisiac effect.

Whilst 'on the bone' meat has not been favoured in Britain lately, for reasons we all know well, its popularity in other countries is still high. Osso Bucco is practically the national meat dish of Italy, though with regional variations. The potency of this dish lies not in the meat which is on the bones, but the bone marrow which lies within them. It is basically a veal leg stew cooked in stock, sometimes chicken, some white wine and peeled and chopped tomatoes. Most Italian restaurants feature this dish, but remember to contain your lust until you get home.

Goat and venison

Goat meat features heavily in ancient recipes and the ram was the symbol of male potency. It is not widely available today, except in the Middle East and Italy. Succulent kid stews, such as that served in the Tuscan restaurant Da Mario, near the Spanish Steps in Rome, have a silky richness which is particularly sensual.

Venison looms large in the history of aphrodisia as the deer and its many relations are inextricably related to male bonding rituals and the lore of the hunt. Dragging back a dead beast was certain to ensure that its killer got a good reception from his women folk. Bringing a haunch or a venison burger from a supermarket does not guarantee the same result, but the fruity flavours of the meat itself will work wonders. It is also, like all game, remarkably fat free. Indeed, it is often necessary to add fat when cooking it, so that it does not dry out. Cook simply and marinade lightly. Often the only thing venison tastes of is the juniper berries which feature too largely in many recipes. Go easy on the juniper, have only a pinch of allspice (details of which are in the following chapter) and, as ever, add whatever spice turns you on. Ginger, perhaps.

Mixed meat loaf

One of the least glamorous dishes, visually and titulary, is Mixed Meat Loaf, but after a few mouthfuls its effects are obvious. Mix together equal quantities of good steak mince and minced venison (mostly available as venison burgers). Add some finely chopped onion, a squeeze of concentrated tomato purée and seasoning, and top with sliced tomato. Put in an oven-proof dish, cover with foil and bake in a medium oven. This is a foolproof dish, so you can forget it is in the oven while engaging in romantic activities!

Hare and rabbit

Hare has many mystical qualities. Images of hares sitting and contemplating the moon, and the Phoenician goddess of love and hunting, Astarte, feature heavily in ancient literature. The traditional dish of Jugged Hare is available in many cookery manuals. Its potency lies in the fact that to make it properly the hare should be cooked in its own blood. It really isn't so difficult, as it is just a stew, in the making of which you have to avoid curdling the blood.

Plain roast or char-grilled hare is best for the squeamish. Take the rack off the bone and cook whole or sliced in medaillons. Braised red cabbage, with apple and sultanas, preferably cooked weeks before and frozen to enhance the flavour, is a perfect accompaniment.

OPPOSITE: MARROW IS THE MAIN APHRODISIAC CONSTITUENT OF OSSO BUCCO.

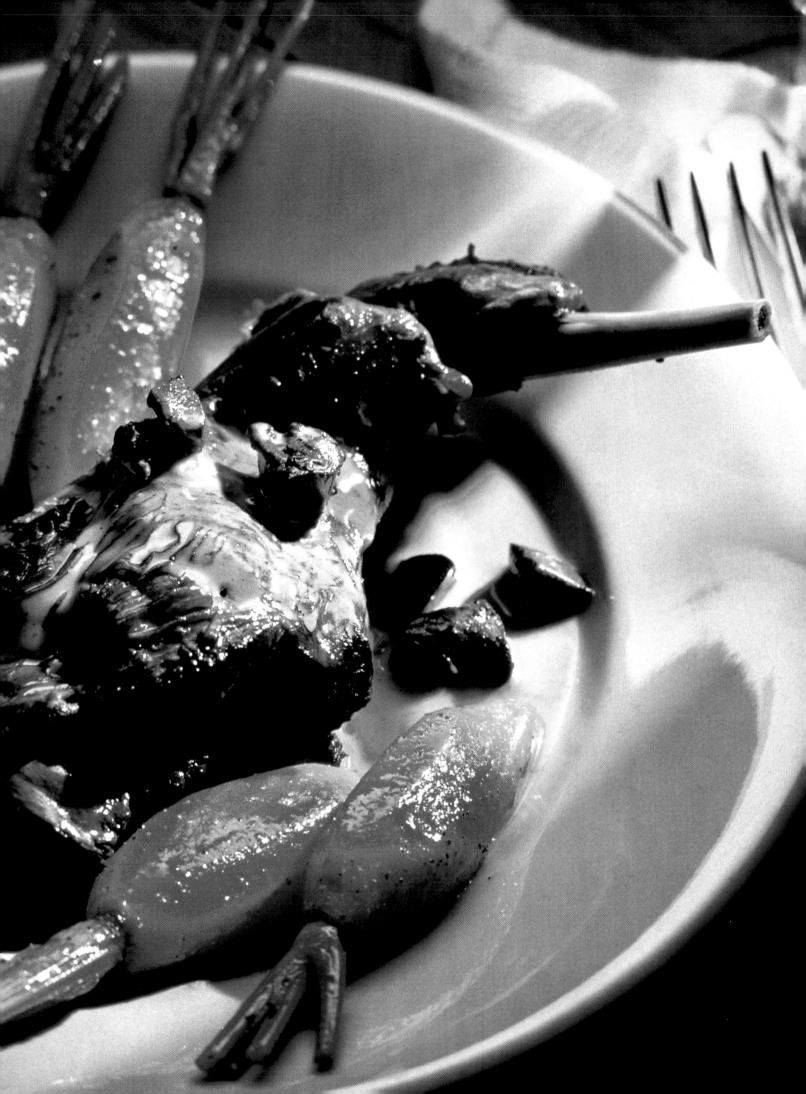

Hare's relation, the rabbit, has less aphrodisiacal effect as it can be bland. The Greeks prepare it best. Chop up a rabbit, or buy a pack of pieces, including the giblets if you wish, and stew in wine with olives, baby onions, peeled, de-seeded and chopped tomatoes, garlic, of course, and some allspice.

Alternatively, if you know your rabbit's recent history (i.e. how fresh it is) marinate the rack and the rear legs in the simplest of marinades and put under a very hot grill until the juices are clear when pierced with a skewer. To hasten the process put the rabbit pieces in the microwave for a minute or two before grilling, or steaming them.

Poultry and game

Feathered friends offer many aphrodisiac opportunities. Even the common chicken. providing you buy free range.

OPPOSITE: HARE IS CONSIDERED TO BE MORE EXOTIC THAN ITS COUSIN THE RABBIT.

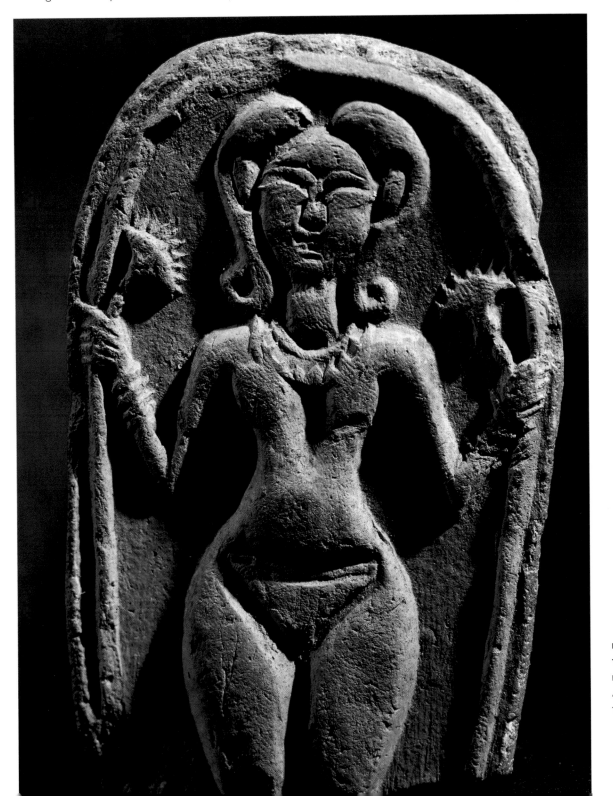

LEFT: ASTARTE, THE MOON GODDESS OF LOVE AND FERTILITY ASSOCIATED WITH THE HARE.

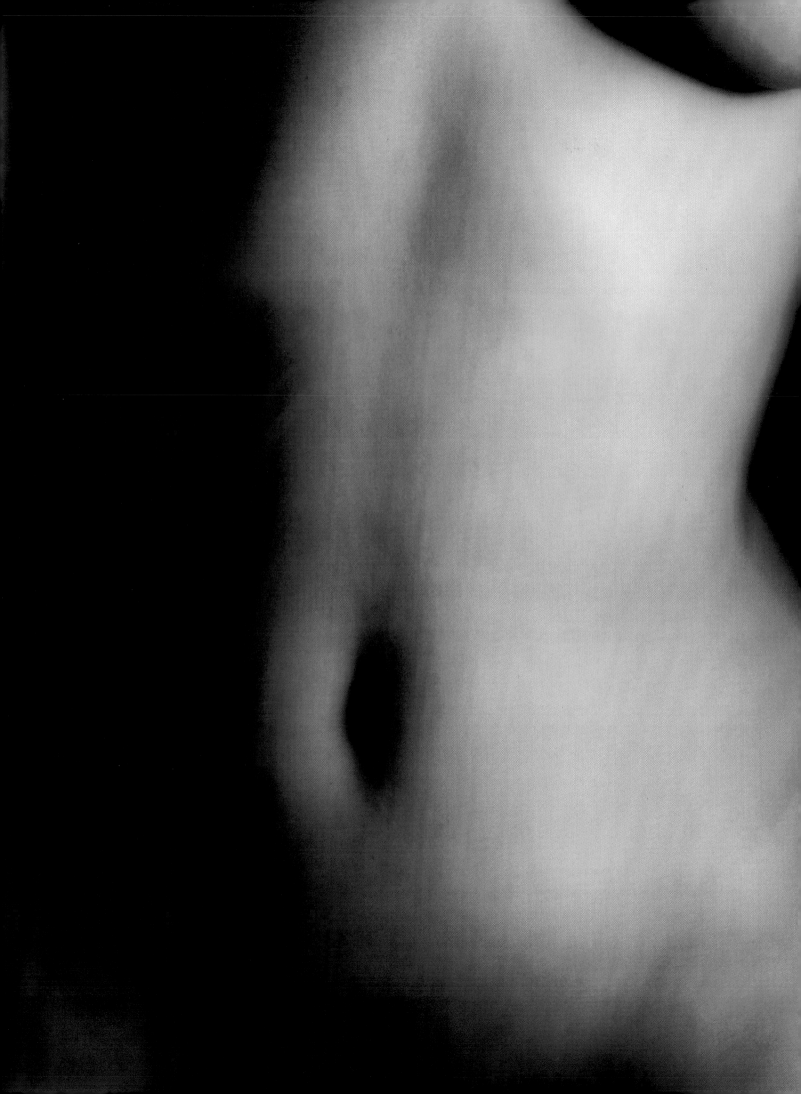

Guinea fowl are recorded even before the chicken we know today, which suggests that they are related to birds the Romans and Greeks knew. One recipe based on old sources is Roast Guinea Fowl with Pomegranate and Thyme. For an intimate dinner for two you will need one guinea fowl and two pomegranates, plus seasoning, including garlic, and some thinly sliced pancetta ham (more refined than bacon) to avoid the bird drying out in roasting. Stuff the bird with the flesh and seeds of one of the pomegranates, some butter, a clove of garlic, some thyme and a slice of the ham. Put the remaining ham slices over the breast and secure with string. Heat some butter in the dish in which you intend to roast the bird. Brown it all over and then place in a medium oven for around half an hour. Baste with some of the juice from the second pomegranate. Roast for a further 15 minutes. Test if the juices run clear between the leg and breast – it may take an extra five minutes. When cooked, take out the bird and allow to rest. Remove any excess fat (there should be little) and add the remaining pomegranate juice to the dish. Reduce for a few minutes until you have a syrupy concoction. Pour over the bird and serve.

Small birds have always attracted those seeking aphrodisiacs. The soaring swallows and migrating sparrows had an allure for the Romans. Sparrows can still be found in Roman street markets and the French still enjoy consuming a selection of migrating birds. For many of the recipes which are handed down we can now substitute reared birds such as the quail, but there is also a ready supply of wild birds such as the pigeon, the partridge and the pheasant, all infinitely superior in flavour, texture and aphrodisiac effect. All are at their best when simply grilled. Cut off the breasts, marinade briefly and then put on a hot griddle, turning once, just long enough to leave a hint of pink. The carcasses and legs can be used to make stocks and game pies.

Pigeon, partridge and pheasant

Pigeon can be simply roasted, with some pancetta ham or smoked bacon on the breasts, with a stuffing of prunes. Pot roasting in red wine, with shallots and a few chopped dried apricots put in towards the end of the cooking produces a luscious meal. Cook on a low heat and for not too long unless you want a shrivelled bird.

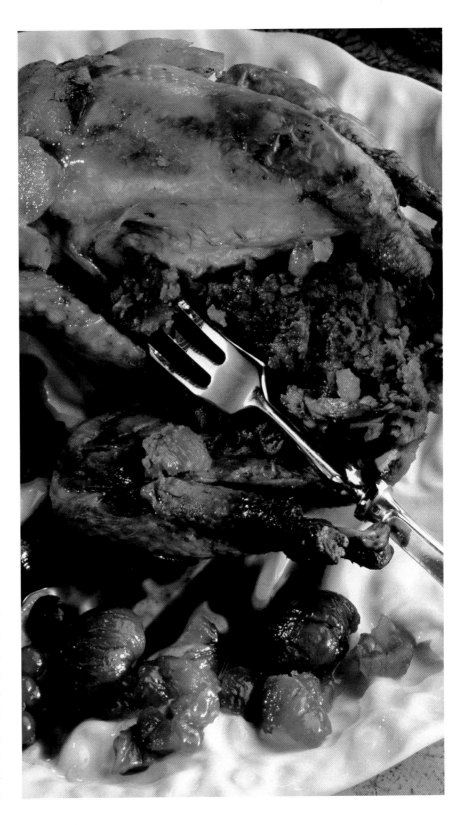

ABOVE: GUINEA FOWL IS A TRULY ANCIENT APHRODISIAC BIRD, SERVED SINCE CLASSICAL TIMES.

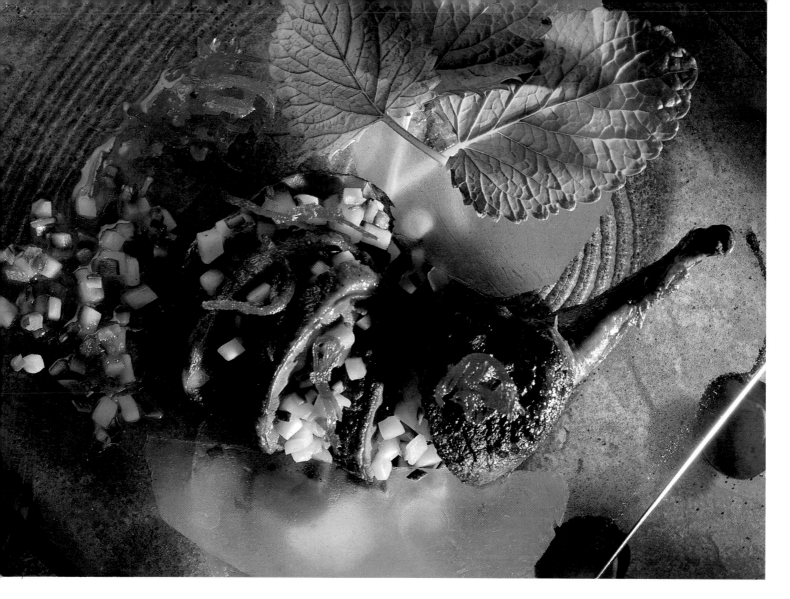

**ABOVE: ANOTHER
ANCIENT DISH – PIGEON,
ADORED BY THE ROMANS.**

The Romans, who liked everything to excess, garnished pigeons with a sauce made from a chopped onion lightly fried in oil, to which mashed dates, some anchovy sauce and pepper were added. The yolks of two eggs should be stirred in carefully (you do not want to end up with scrambled eggs) followed by a good spoonful each of honey and wine vinegar. The amounts of the last two can be adjusted to suit your own sweet and sour taste. Simmer for a short while to allow the flavours to combine. A few roughly torn leaves of celery or coriander can be strewn on top.

Partridges are delicate by most game standards and are best simply roasted, with considerable basting, in a fairly high oven for a short time. Don't let them dry out. A good moist stuffing helps and, as with so many birds, roasting them on their sides for part of the time helps the juices infuse the breast. For a seasonal twist, peel a small pear a couple of days in advance and soak in Armagnac. Sprinkle with cinnamon or allspice and

**OPPOSITE: PHEASANT
IS A RICH-TASTING
WOODLAND BIRD.**

insert into the bird. Brown the bird, put in your casserole with some shallots. When the shallots start to colour, add a dash more Armagnac and enough water to keep the bird moist. Another 30 or so minutes should suffice, but check that the juices between leg and breast run clear. If you wish to play the ace, and cholesterol is no problem to you, stir some double cream into the juices until they thicken. Console yourself with the knowledge that much of the alcohol content will have evaporated.

Pheasants can be treated in much the same way. Again they have very lean meat with that wonderful taste of the woods. They have the same richness as other birds, which can only be called gamey, a word which in itself has sexual connotations.

Goose

The Ancient Greeks and Romans celebrated the goose in much the same way as the Chinese celebrated the pig, eating every part of it. It can be roasted just like

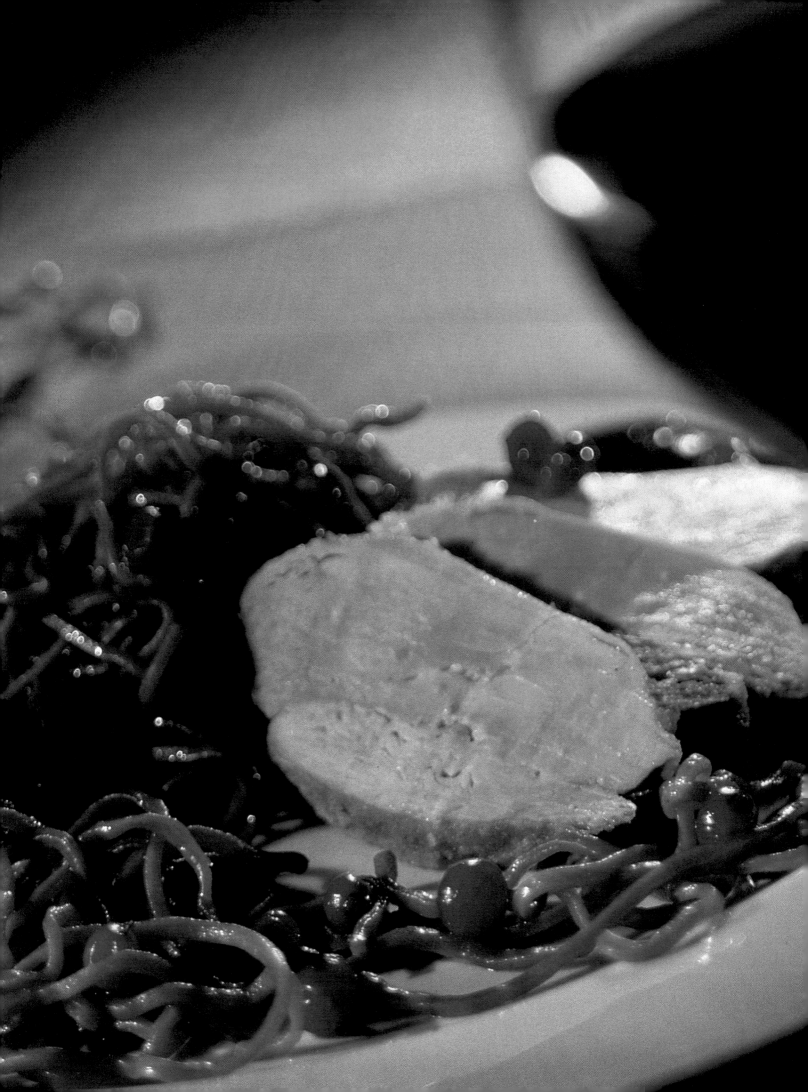

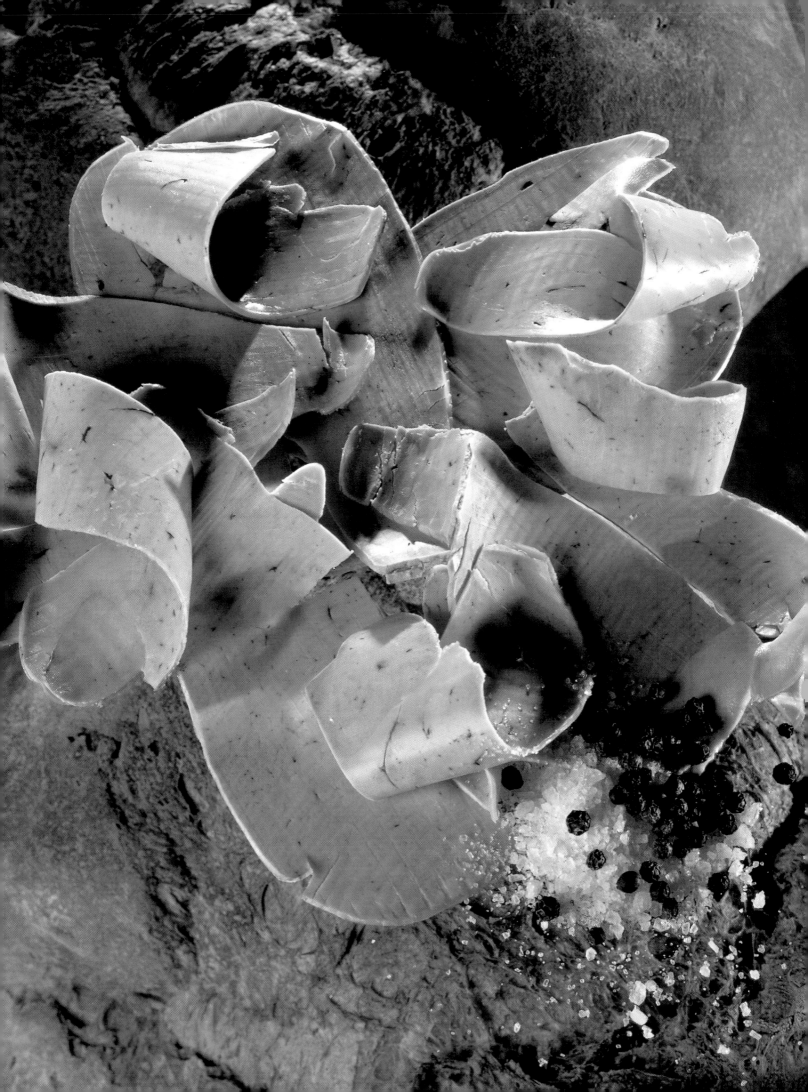

other birds, except that it does not need added fat. In fact, it produces prodigious amounts that has to be constantly siphoned off. Leaving the bird in a chilly place, with a pricked breast, for some days before roasting, can help crisp up the skin. The resulting fat can be stored to use in the making of perfect roast potatoes. Goose is rich and can only be improved by adding other richly aphrodisiac ingredients. Stuff with a mixture of chestnuts and prunes, perhaps with a chopped apple to cut through the richness.

The goose's greatest contribution to aphrodisia, at some considerable detriment to itself, is undeniably foie gras. This is one of the great aphrodisiacs, alongside the truffle, garlic and oysters. If you are adventurous, and you should be in matters of the heart, make your own foie gras. Buy a large, skinned goose liver. Marinate in Cognac, salt and pepper for 24 hours. Use a terrine, into which the liver fits tightly. Slice it down the middle and insert thinly sliced truffle. Cover with pork fat and cook in a bain-marie in a medium oven for about 35 minutes. Don't let the water in the bain-marie boil. Allow to chill before serving. You can, of course, buy foie gras in a jar, or a tin, from a delicatessen. Wherever you obtain it, it is worth the expense and effort of purchasing, even if only once or twice a year. As it is expensive and therefore scarce, duck livers can be substituted, but is the economy worth it? Traditionally it is served with a Sauternes wine jelly, made by dissolving a leaf of gelatine in a good Sauternes, allowing it to set and then chopping roughly. Foie gras can also be used in an extravagant dish, ideal for that special occasion, if you happen to like offal.

Sweetbreads are an acquired taste, a little going a long way, as they are so rich and creamy. The foreplay includes simmering the sweetbreads in water, with a bayleaf, and onion, a clove and some carrot, the day before you intend to serve the dish. After half an hour, let the liquid cool. Peel the skin from the sweetbreads and flatten them by placing under a flat dish weighed down, for a few hours. On the day you intend to deploy this dish cut them into portions, and dust lightly with seasoned flour. Fry in butter for 10 to 15 minutes, until they are golden outside and firm inside, but not hard. Put in a warm place with a sliver of truffle on

each piece. Then, in the juices they have left, fry whatever pieces of truffle you can afford, together with finely sliced shallots. Add some dry white wine and some chicken stock and bubble with a knob or two of butter to make a shiny sauce. Take out the slivers of truffle before the final burst of bubbling. Scatter over the sweetbreads and serve.

The love of liver is not an accident, for the Ancients believed that the basic life-force of the body came from the liver and not the heart as we now know. This is why it was regarded as such an important sexual stimulant. Pliny wrote that the ultimate was eagle's liver, but that is hardly a realistic ingredient today.

Other ideas

Other oddities to some cultures, but close to the heart of others, include snails. Most authorities consider that

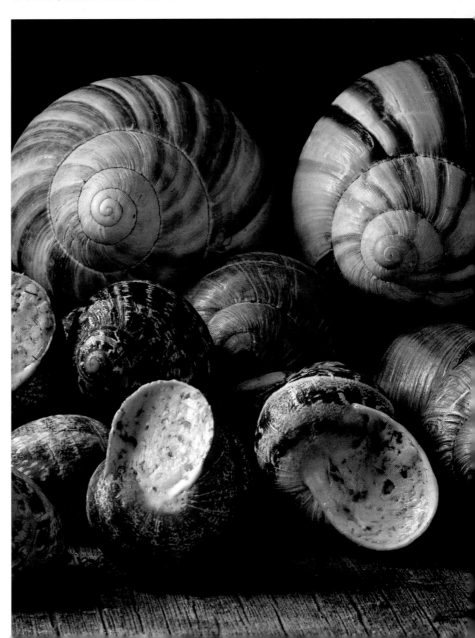

the snail is not intrinsically aphrodisiac, but that it is the rich garlic and butter sauce they come with. Ancient lore has it that they resemble female genitalia and are therefore aphrodisiacal. They do, however, have a high mineral content, which can stimulate. And, once again, the act of eating them is highly suggestive.

Dismembered frog is also an unenticing prospect, but providing you only have to deal with pristine, skinned and sautéed legs, they are highly regarded, particularly in France. Once again the liquid in which they are cooked; good oil, butter, wine and lashings of garlic, adds to the effect.

The last oddity of the ancients, still much-prized today, is Bird's Nest Soup. The nests are retrieved from caves where a species of swallow builds its nest from sea algae, pasted together with their saliva. They are cleaned, pressed and then sold in small quantities for large sums throughout the Far East. They are then simmered to make an aromatic soup. Like Mock Turtle soup, the most readily available is in tins and can be but a pale imitation of the original concoction.

An Ambrosial Interlude

Most aphrodisiacs act as stimulants, but honey is also one of the best and fastest-acting sources of revitalising energy. There can only be frustration if you are stimulated and aroused, yet are too tired to perform sexually. Though most people obtain sufficient energy from their regular meals, there are many situations where a more immediate surge of energy is needed.

Honey is a healer as well as a stimulant and energy provider. An Egyptian papyrus of medical lore going back well over three thousand years lists close to a thousand remedies and in over half of them honey features. Symbolically, honey itself defies decay and seems to have eternal life. In the ancient ruins of Paestum in Italy, archaeologists unearthed an urn of honey. It was still as golden and sticky as it had been some two and a half thousand years ago, when it was buried in the tomb.

The effects of honey are easier to quantify than many other potential aphrodisiacs. In sexual activity, as in sport, blood sugar is used up more quickly than usual. The more vigorous the activity, the quicker the level of blood sugar falls. Eating everyday foods will bring the level back to normal, but only after a time. This is when honey plays its part, by providing a quick 'fix'. Unlike other instant energy providers, such as glucose, honey has absolutely no side effects. It works equally well for both young and old.

It is no accident that in the many treatises on sexual activity from Arabia, the legendary land of sexual prowess, sweetmeats made from honey were always recommended. And they were always at hand. The Arabian physician and philosopher Avicena suggested a mixture of honey, pepper and ginger for instant effect. Further east, it would be true to say that without those dishes of honey and spices, the *Kama Sutra* might never have been written.

Honey also counteracts the effects of alcohol, which is why it is advisable to eat a honey-based sweet after a romantic dinner, if you want the romance to blossom perfectly. A spoonful or two of honey taken before the meal will also line the stomach, preventing the absorption of too much alcohol.

There is a multitude of recipes involving honey. It can be used to glaze meats, enrich sauces or bind together fruity concoctions. Many will be found in this book.

HONEY – HEALER, STIMULANT AND ENERGY PROVIDER.

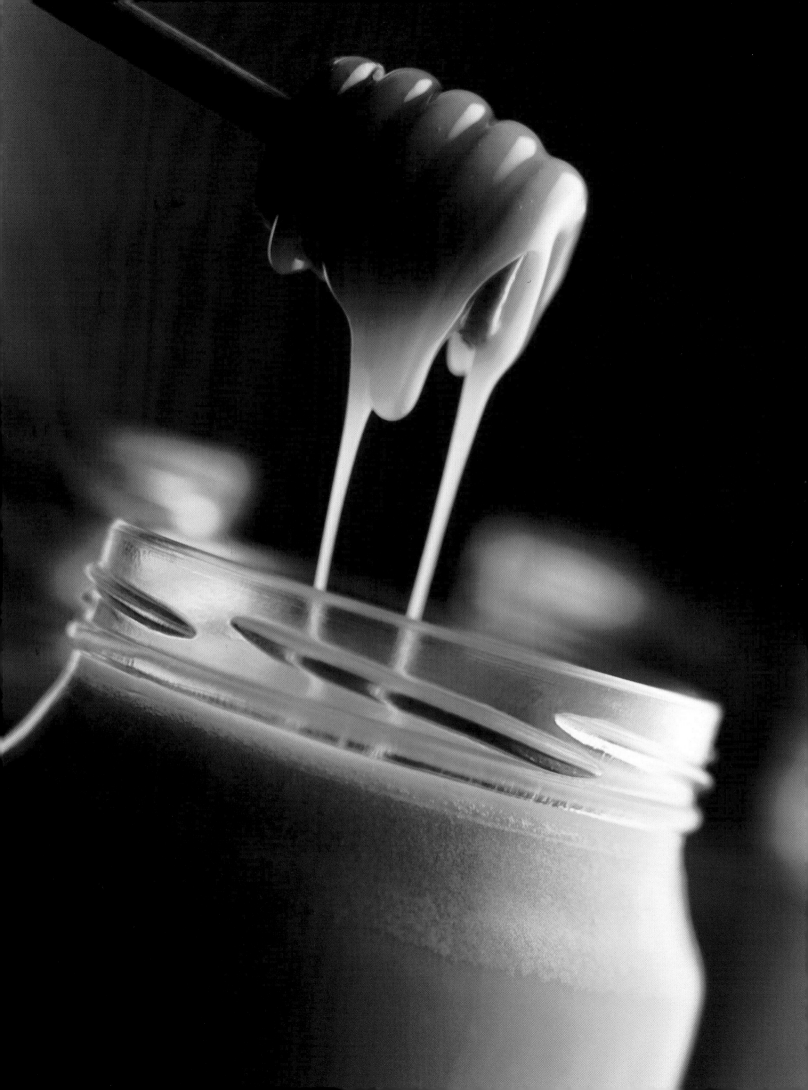

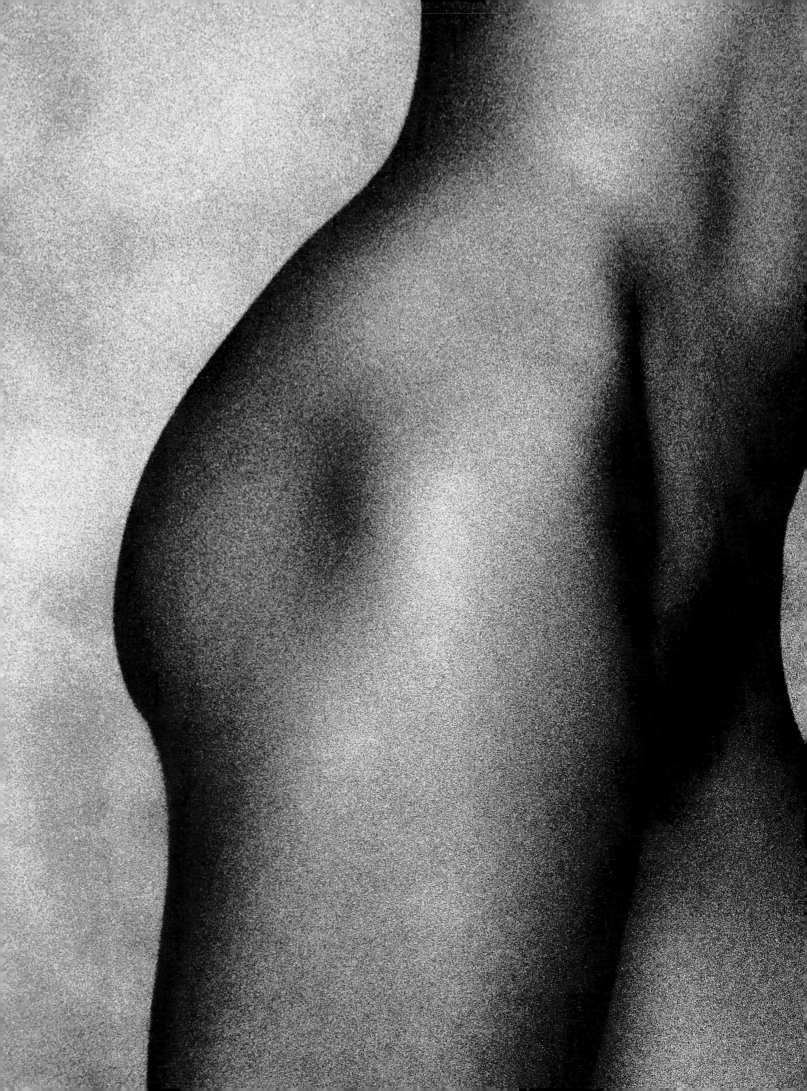

5

SPICE UP YOUR LOVE LIFE

The herbs and spices we use today are almost exactly the same as those which appear in Greek, Roman, Arabic and Eastern literature, and this includes their aphrodisiac properties. We can therefore draw on many centuries of knowledge in our search for spices with very special aphrodisiac qualities.

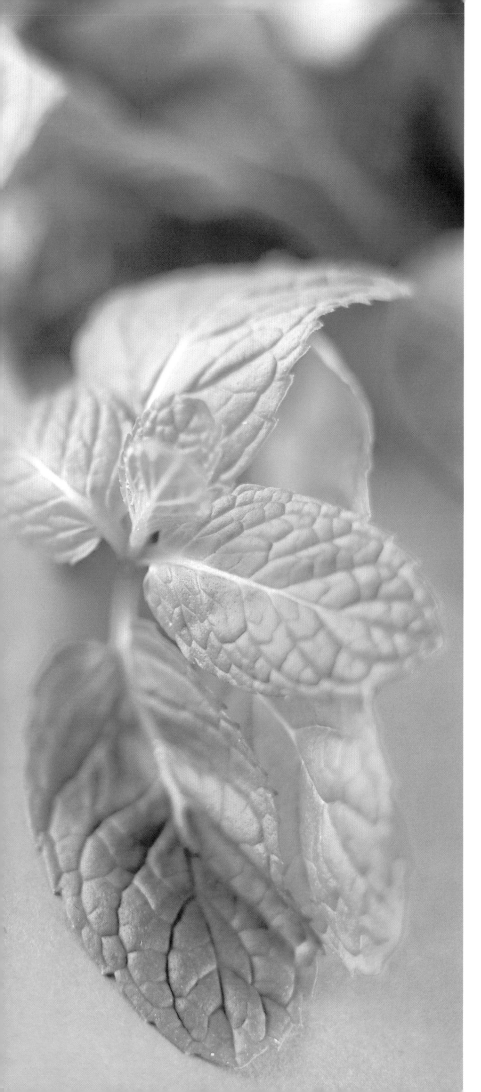

Herbs

One of the earliest recorded herbs to be used is fennel, the stalk of which, Sophocles claimed, was used by Prometheus to bring the spark of fire to Earth from Olympus. The seeds were said to give strength and long life. Charlemagne planted it in his herb garden and it was used on fast days to dull the appetite. It is related to the Anise family and has similar properties and flavour. Anise seeds allegedly excited the passions of newlyweds, either in the form of syrups or liqueurs. The French use it as a basis for pastis, the Greek for ouzo and the Turkish for raki – aphrodisiac drinks for passionate nations.

Mint is a highly regarded aphrodisiac. Shakespeare wrote of it as a stimulant for middle-aged gentlemen. Its refreshing coolness makes it an excellent balance to warmth-inducing spices. It is one of the most common herbs and grows like a weed. It is particularly favoured as a strong, heavily-sugared tea in the Middle East.

An unusual chutney accompaniment for a hot curry involves a good bunch of mint, a small onion, a spoonful of honey and a small peeled apple. Blend together, then season with a little salt and a pinch of hot cayenne pepper.

Another delicate aphrodisiac way to use mint is as Sugared Mint Leaves. Pick the best undamaged mint leaves. Paint on both sides with slightly beaten egg white and evenly coat with castor sugar. Leave to dry in a warm place, such as an airing cupboard.

Parsley has a varied history as an aphrodisiac, because of its association with the Devil and witchcraft. As it is slow to germinate is was said to 'go seven times to the Devil and back', and it was allegedly made into a paste by witches to help them fly.

Today, we know it to be full of vitamins and minerals which envigorate the blood and organs. It is best taken plain as a garnish to a main course, as part of a salad or, one of the most common ways, as parsley butter to

LEFT: MINT IS
REGARDED AS A
STIMULANT FOR
MIDDLE-AGED MEN.

RIGHT: THYME,
A HIGHLY AROMATIC
APHRODISIAC HERB.

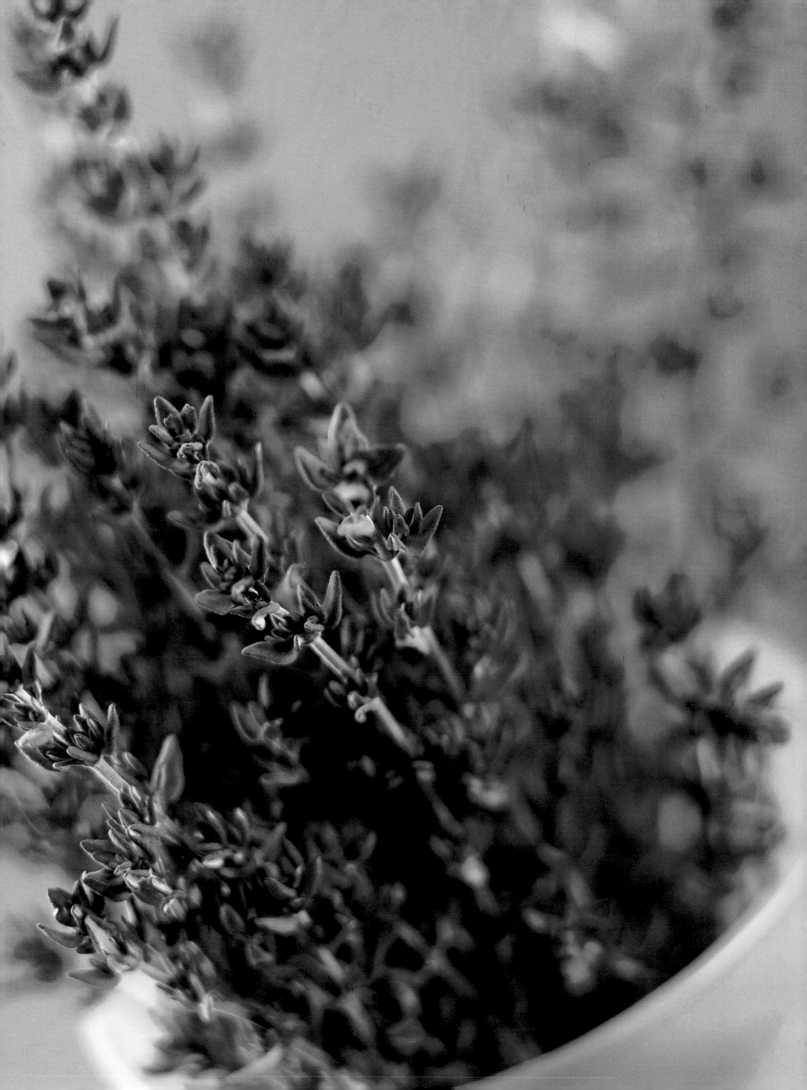

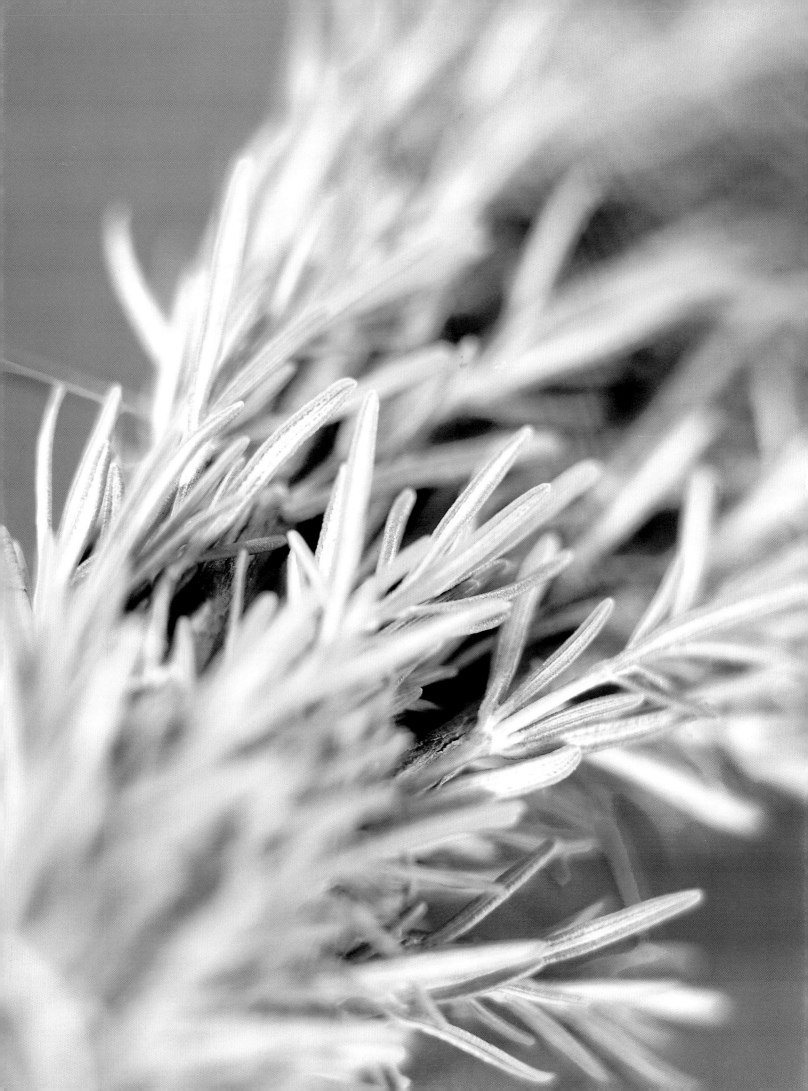

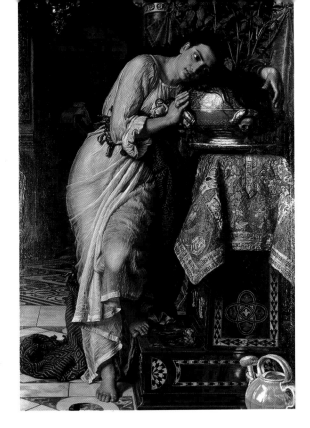

serve with grilled meat and fish. This is simply made by mashing finely chopped parsley in the butter with a few drops of lemon juice.

Chervil has many of the properties of parsley and is another prolific grower. It has been recorded as an aphrodisiac since Tudor times.

Basil is for many the king of herbs, indeed, it takes its name from the Greek basileus, meaning 'king'. Hence, in France, it is known as the Herbe Royale. Culpeper writes that 'it makes a man merrie and glad'. It is the symbol of fecundity and passion in many cultures, including the voodoo worshippers of Haiti. In his *Decameron*, Boccaccio told the story of the young noblewoman, Isabella, whose lover was beheaded by her brothers. She buried the head in a pot of basil, which naturally flourished. John Keats wrote an epic poem on the same subject

Basil should only be used when fresh and then only added to hot dishes at the very end of cooking. Its aroma is sensual in itself, creating instantly the aura of the sun-drenched countries of the Mediterranean region.

One of the most popular uses of basil is in the Italian pesto sauce. This can be made at home, but it takes a lot of basil, so buying good quality ready-made jars is more convenient. It consists of basil leaves pounded to a paste, together with garlic, a little salt and some pine nuts. Grated parmesan cheese is then added

with olive oil. Use as a simple sauce over a favourite pasta, as a pizza topping or as a coating for grilled chicken breast.

Chives are not strictly speaking a herb, but are mostly used as a garnish or in a salad dish. They are a member of the onion family and are related to garlic, which gives them a bonus in the aphrodisiac stakes. They are often popular with those who don't like pungent garlic. They should always be used freshly cut and added to any warm dish at the last minute. They are excellent in omelettes.

Sage is a strong herb which should be used in moderation, especially as it is a potent stimulant for fertility. In Ancient Greece, it is written that wives welcomed returning soldiers home with sage tea to encourage sexual advances. Culpeper thought that it 'is singular good for quickening the senses' which could help in amorous situations. It is best used as garnish, as sauce or in pot roasts involving game meats.

OPPOSITE: ROSEMARY
FOR REMEMBRANCE.

LEFT: *ISABELLA AND
THE POT OF BASIL*, BY
WILLIAM HOLMAN HUNT.

BELOW: BASIL,
CONSIDERED THE KING
OF HERBS BY MANY.

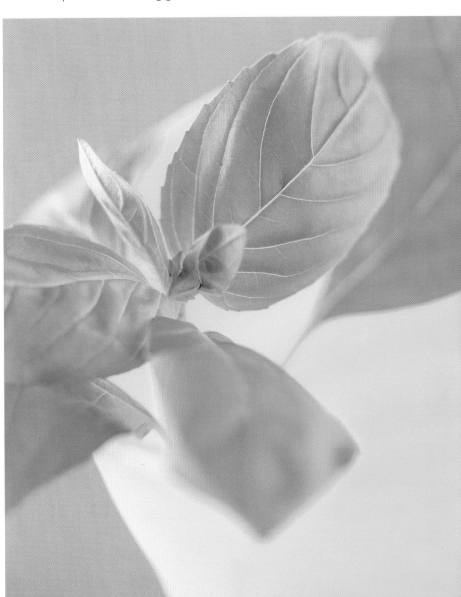

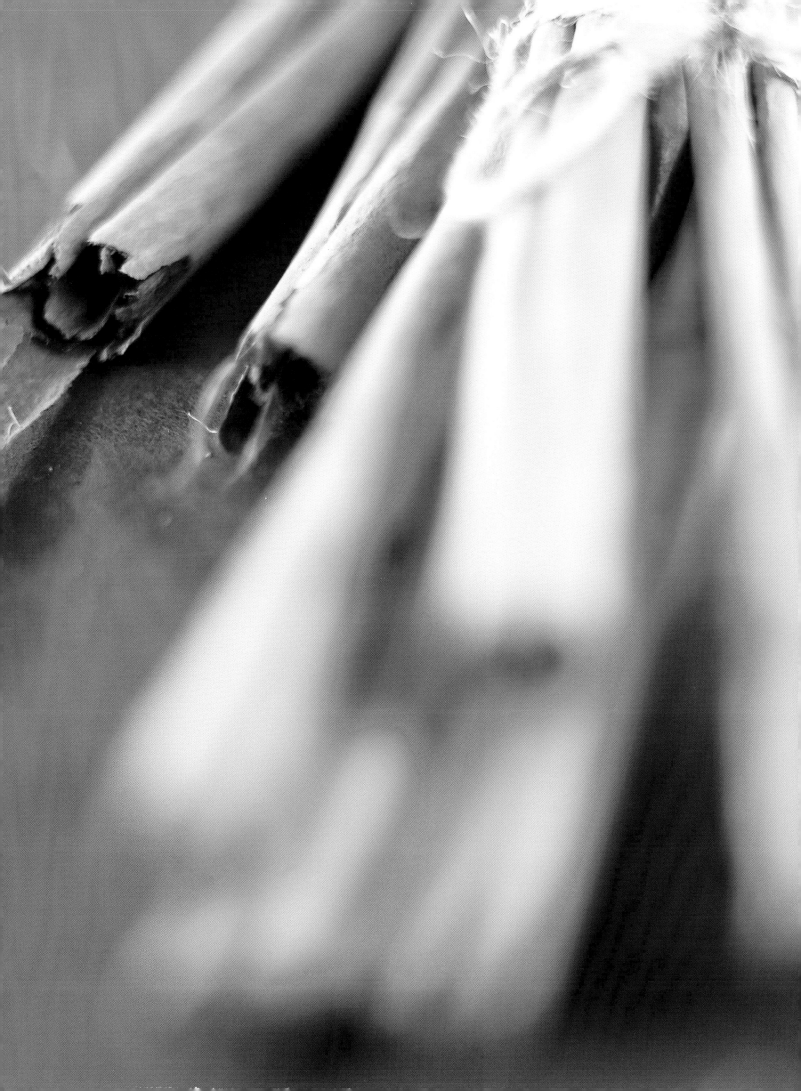

Other ideas

In general, all herbs are good for you, particularly those previously described. Others include dill, popularly believed to be an aphrodisiac by the Scandinavians. Its most efficacious use is in the preparation of marinaded salmon, known as gravad lax, now readily available in supermarkets. Thyme is mostly effective through its aroma, oregano has a penetrating flavour redolent of the Mediterranean, whilst coriander is best when used as seeds in casseroles or as torn leaves to garnish a curry. Its sweet scent, with a hint of oranges, evokes the mysterious Orient, which always encourages romance.

Two spiky plants are effective aphrodisiacs, rosemary and lavender. Rosemary is one of the most pungent herbs and is best used when inserted into roasts, particularly lamb. It is not high on the aphrodisiac scale, but creates a heady aroma. It also increases the blood flow, aiding stimulation.

Lavender was highly regard in the Middle Ages, but is only now making a comeback in the kitchen. An infusion of lavender can be used to make an aromatic sorbet and sprigs can be added to stews such as rabbit and veal. As with rosemary the sprigs should be removed before serving and the liquid strained to make sure no spears have come free. If you are not keen on lavender in the kitchen, a lavender bag beneath the pillow creates a pleasant aroma.

As with herbs, some spices merely add scent and flavour to a dish, while others enjoy serious reputations as aphrodisiacs.

Allspice is also known as Jamaican pepper, as it is a dried, ground berry which comes mainly from the West Indies. It is a single spice, but is reminiscent of cloves, cinnamon and nutmeg. Apart from its use in stews and soups it can also be used to make a tempting dessert known as Sweet 'n Spice. Add icing sugar to a stiffly beaten egg white which has been mixed with a teaspoon of allspice and some rose water. Roll the mixture out and cut into suggestive shapes. Leave to harden in a low oven with the door open. These make suggestive titbits to end a meal with.

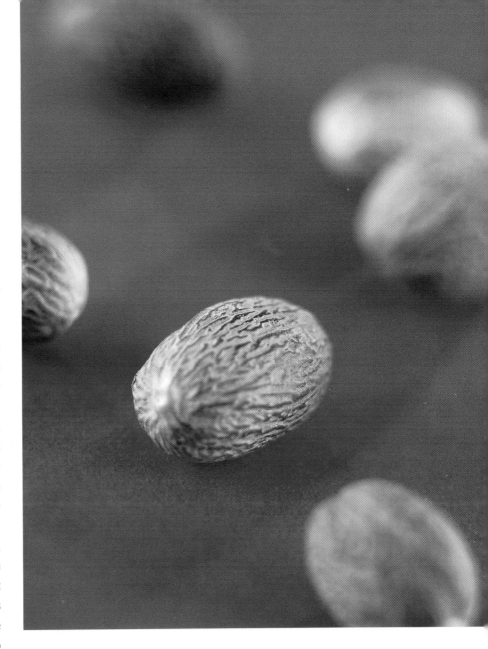

ABOVE: WHOLE NUTMEGS.

Spice up your love life

Cinnamon is one of the oldest recorded aphrodisiac spices. It comes from the inner bark of the cinnamon tree and is best used as rolled sticks, though the powdered form is more common and more convenient for use in baking. It is very versatile, being used in curry powders, in baked apples and apple pies, to flavour tea and coffee or as an essential ingredient of warming mulled wine.

Nutmeg and mace come from the same tree, mace being the bright red covering of the hard seed, which is the nutmeg. A drink containing the two spices was traditionally given to bridegrooms in the Middle Ages to give them added vigour. Nutmeg is best used freshly grated as it loses its flavour quickly. Miniature grinders are sold, to accommodate the acorn-like nut. The uses of nutmeg and mace are much the same as those of cinnamon.

OPPOSITE: STICKS OF
SPICY CINNAMON.

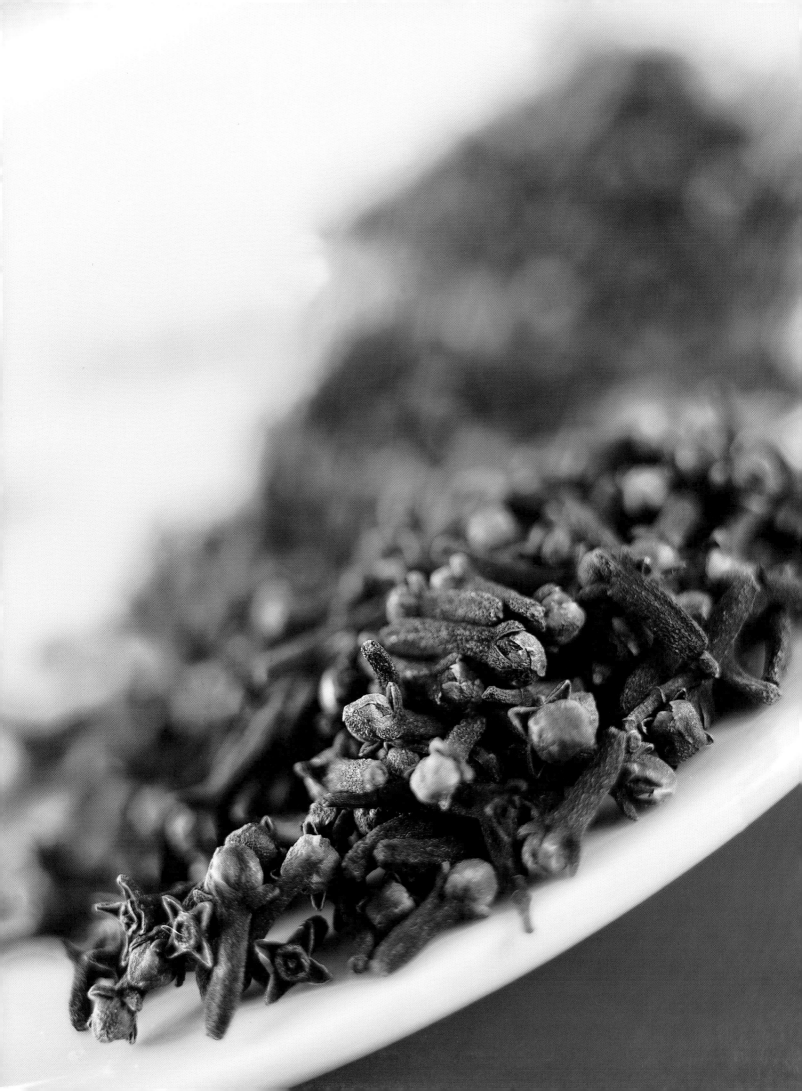

Cloves are a middle range aphrodisiac, reminiscent of cosy winter evenings spent around a real fire, near which hangs a pomander – an orange studded with cloves. It is another ingredient of mulled wine and imparts warm flavours when used to marinate rich meats such as venison, or to spike the skin of a large roast ham.

Ginger is one of the kings of aphrodisia and one of the most versatile. It can be used in sweet or savoury dishes, or eaten on its own when crystallised – preferably coated with chocolate. A true stimulant. Jamaican ginger is of the highest quality and, reputedly, the most effective. Raw, finely grated ginger is the traditional accompaniment to the Japanese raw fish dishes, sushi and sashimi – powerful aphrodisiacs in their own right.

A sensual end to a meal is the combination of the warmth of ginger with the chill of ice. Beat four egg yolks in 250 ml of milk, then mix in 500g of white sugar and two teaspoons of fine powdered ginger. Heat slowly and stir in a double boiler until the mixture thickens. Allow to cool and then chill, but don't freeze.

Winter Warmer

Many spices are brought together to create a traditional, warm winter drink; mulled wine in Britain, glühwein in Germany and Austria, or vin chaud in France. To make a hot winter drink, first spike an orange and an apple with cloves. Slice a second orange. Place all in some moderately good red wine, together with some cinnamon, some freshly ground nutmeg and sugar to taste. Heat up slowly for about 15 minutes, but do not allow to boil. After it has simmered, add a dash of brandy to replace some of the alcohol which has been lost in the simmering. Serve hot.

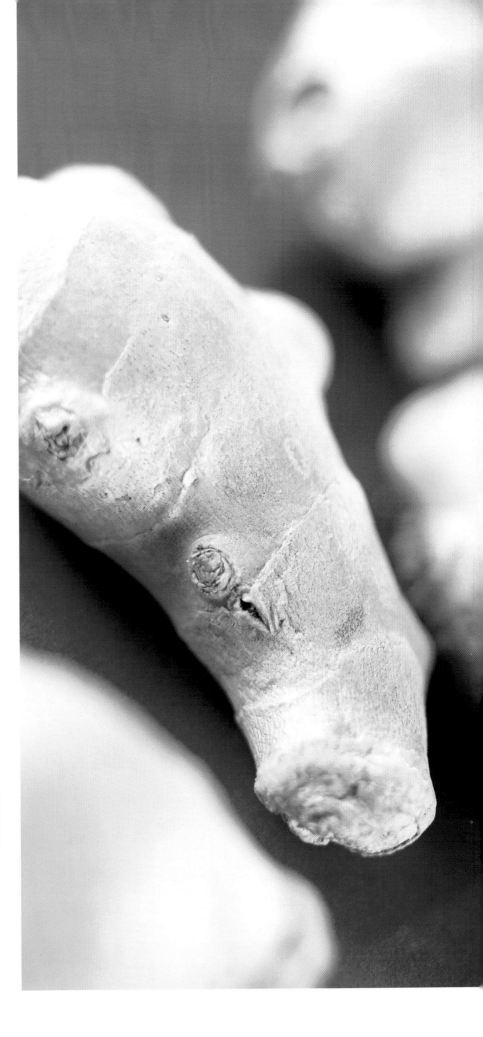

LEFT: CLOVES
CAN PROVIDE A
RICH AMBIENCE
OF FLAVOURS.

RIGHT:
GINGER BRINGS
WARMTH TO
RELATIONSHIPS.

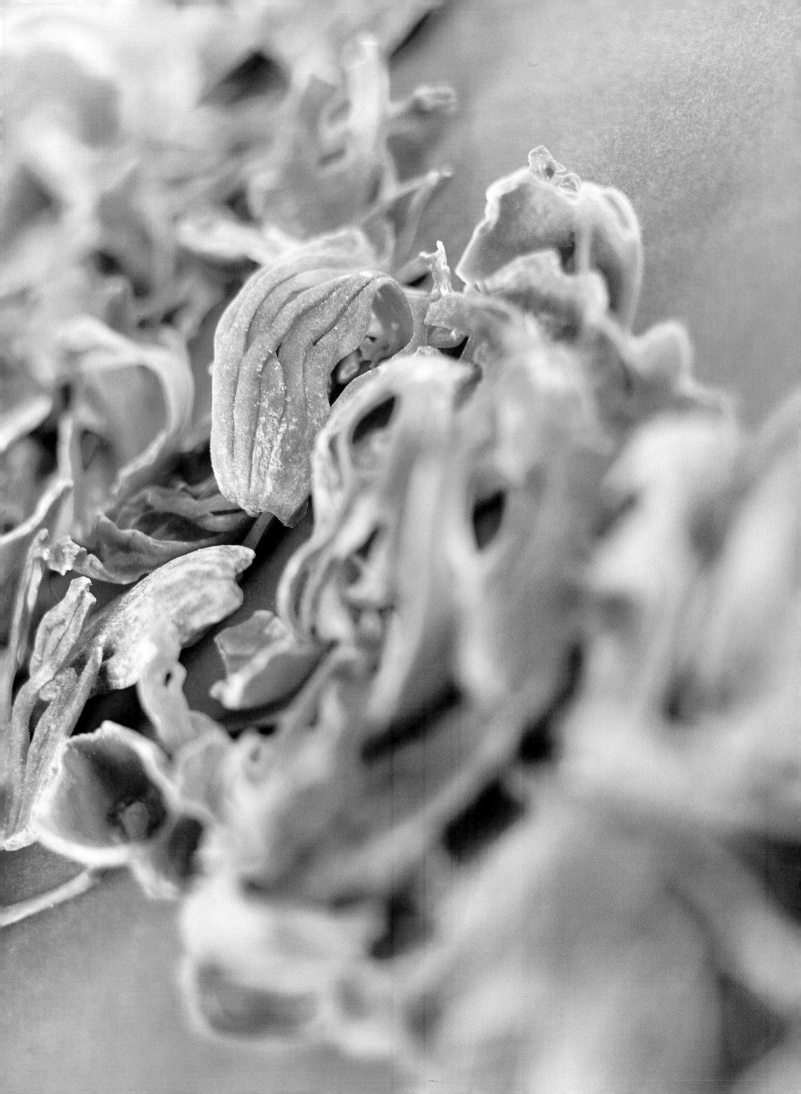

To help this down try Gingerbread with Honey, to end a romantic dinner. Thin 125g of honey with 300ml of hot water or milk. Add 125g sugar, one teaspoon of bicarbonate of soda and one teaspoon of ground aniseed and ginger. Combine in a bowl and slowly add 250g of sifted flour. Butter a cake tin and dust with flour. Bake in a hot oven, gas mark 6 (400F, 200C) for an hour, or until a knife inserted in the middle comes out clean.

Ginger is also an essential ingredient of a very sensual dessert, Cosway Pears. It is used alongside the main aphrodisiac element, cardamom, which is a highly perfumed pod, reminiscent of Arabia, but originally from India. To make Cosway Pears, allow one good-sized pear per person. Peel, retaining the stalk. Poach in enough white wine to cover them, together with the juice and zest of an orange, a cinnamon stick, some ground ginger and two or three cardamom pods per pear. When tender, remove from the liquid. Add sugar to the wine and bubble gently until it makes a syrup. Serve the pears in individual goblets, with the syrup poured over. Honey gingerbread can be used to mop up the aromatic syrup.

Hot stuff

The final group of spices to hot up your love life include the families of peppers, mustards and chillies. On the aphrodisiac scale mustard comes first. Plain English mustard, in versatile powder form is bright yellow and very hot. French mustards are, in general, a warm brown and more aromatic. Mustard seeds can be sprinkled on all manner of dishes, or used to make pickles. It is hardly ever worth the effort of making your own mustard, as there is such a plethora of types available. If you do, take some black mustard seeds and grind them. Add sufficient, good white wine vinegar to make a paste. You can then create your own mustard by adding your favourite ingredients. A little honey will help bind it, followed by ground chilli or ginger for heat, cinnamon or

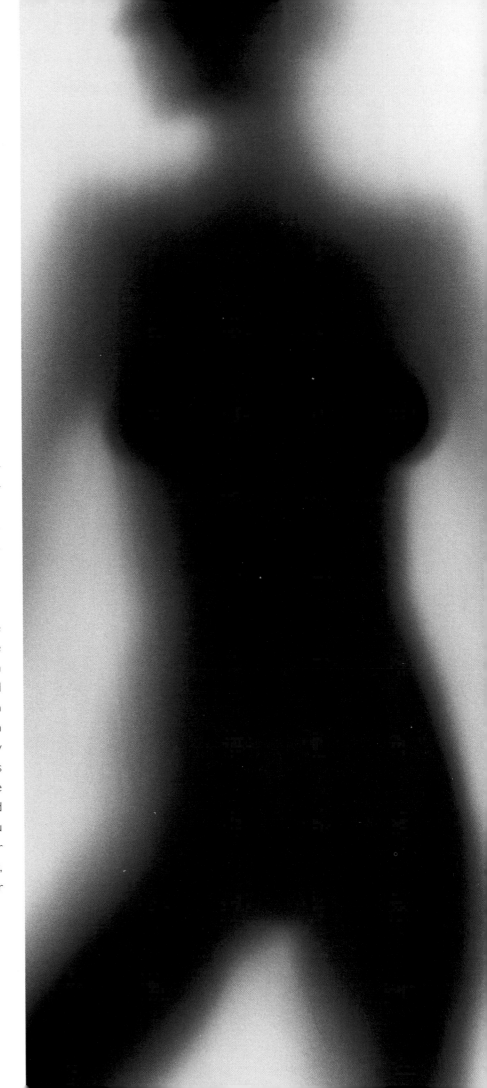

LEFT: MACE IS EXTRACTED FROM THE SAME TREE AS NUTMEG.

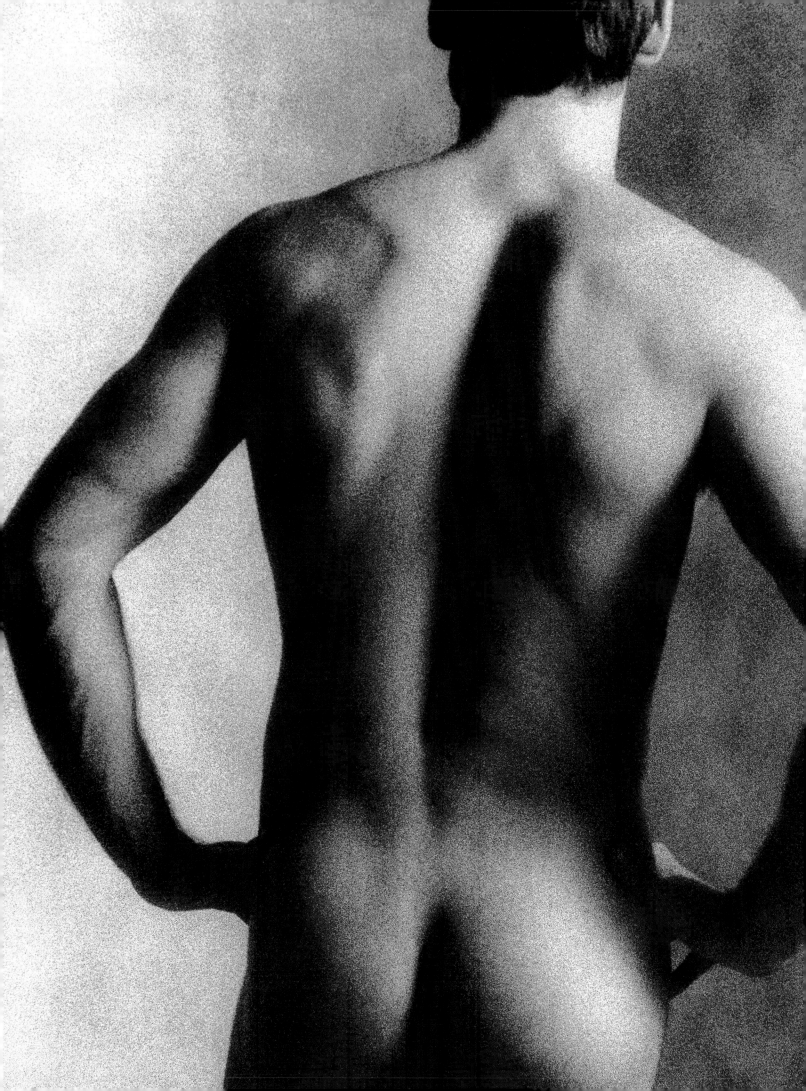

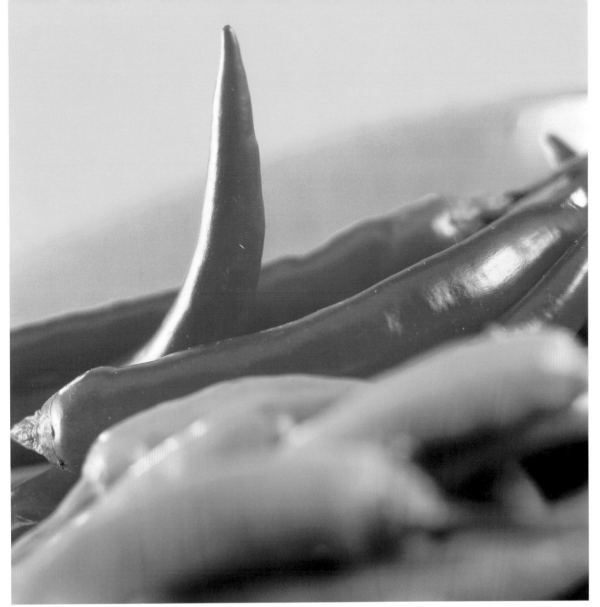

turmeric for flavour, dill or coriander for more exotic effects. There are many more variations you can try.

Chillies are the next most potent aphrodisiac, but must be treated with caution. You may end up inflamed, in quite the wrong way. If overused the chilli heat will overpower other flavours in a dish. Wherever possible use fresh, whole chillies, and remove them before serving. Chilli powder is best avoided, as it is too easy to over-season, and a 'powdery' taste often lingers. The only powdered version used regularly is the lethally hot cayenne pepper, which is manufactured from ground, red peppers. Use sparingly.

Saffron is regarded by many as one of the supreme aphrodisiacs and it still benefits from the Law of Rarity. In other words, it is still very expensive. The saffron we use is made from the pistils of the saffron crocus, which flourished near the town of Saffron Walden, in England. Its flavour is subtle, its golden-red colour infusing dishes with the ultimate luscious aura.

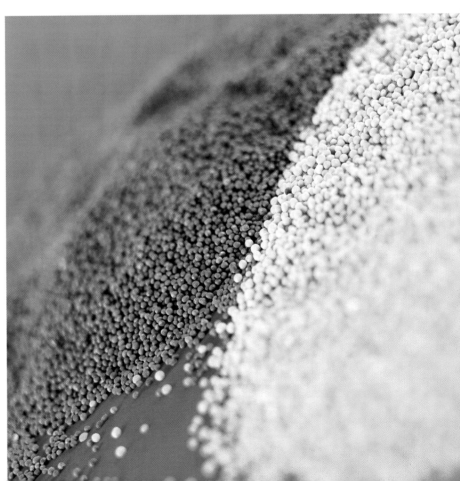

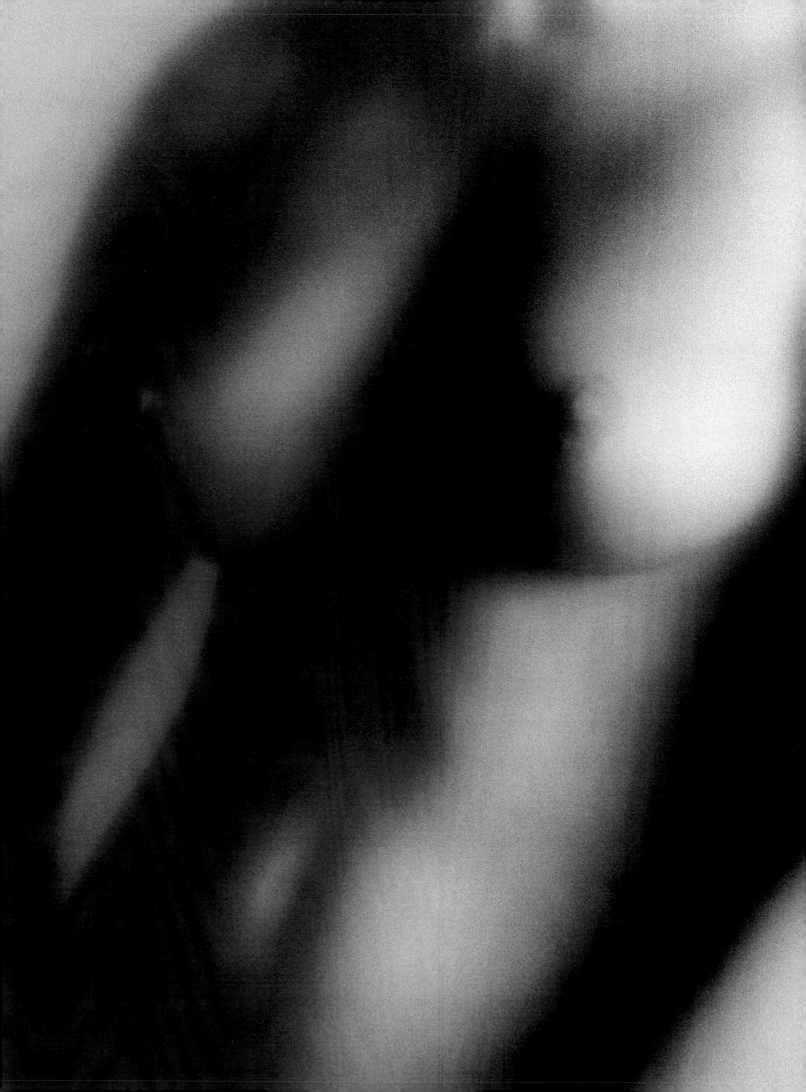

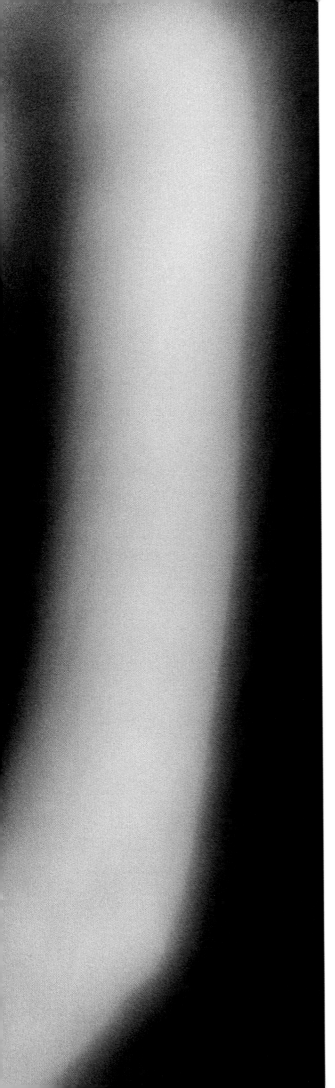

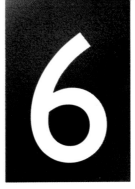

FRUITS OF ORCHARD AND VINE

It is not surprising that many fruits are associated with aphrodisia. In the Bible, Eve used a fruit to lead Adam into temptation. It is highly likely, though, that the apple depicted in so many paintings as the symbol of temptation was originally depicted as an apricot. But the bright red apple has become synonymous with temptation, from the earliest religious paintings to Walt Disney's Snow White.

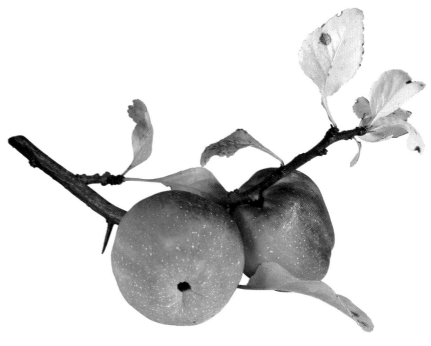

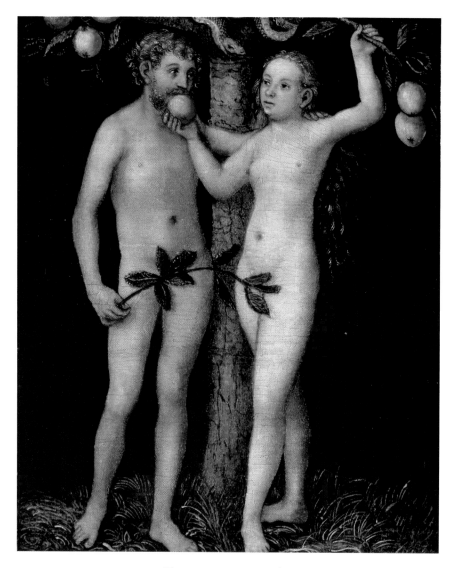

Eastern exotica

The quince has a well-established place in the history of aphrodisia. The 'marmalo' made from this fruit was probably the precursor of today's marmalade. It played an essential role in wedding feasts as it was one of the symbolic fruits of Aphrodite, goddess of love (and sexual fulfilment).

The pomegranate is associated with the apple and the quince, again through Aphrodite. It is a fruit of the erotic Middle East, where it was imbued with much symbolism. It was associated with fertility and its seeds were scattered during wedding festivities. In Greece, it was also part of drunken Dionysian orgies. Its properties are now being recognised once more. Pomegranate molasses from the Bekha valley in Lebanon is now available from top-class supermarkets, to use as a marinade,

a salad dressing or to dribble over ice cream. It is tart and sweet. A pomegranate evening, truly aphrodisiacal, could start with your favourite salad leaves with the pomegranate dressing, then going on to the previously-described Guinea Fowl with Pomegranate and ending with pomegranate sorbet; a good champagne or mild lemon sorbet, mushed together with a little pomegranate molasses and returned to the freezer for a short time. You can, of course, start from scratch. There are many basic recipes.

It's a date

Dates are also rich in trace elements, vitamins and calories, all of which enhance sexual performance. It can be no accident that they originate in the Middle East. A few dates can supply the energy of a whole meal, thus leaving the diner with the extra energy for whatever sensual pleasure is planned. If you intend to

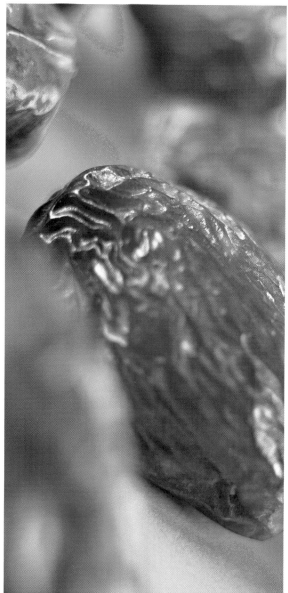

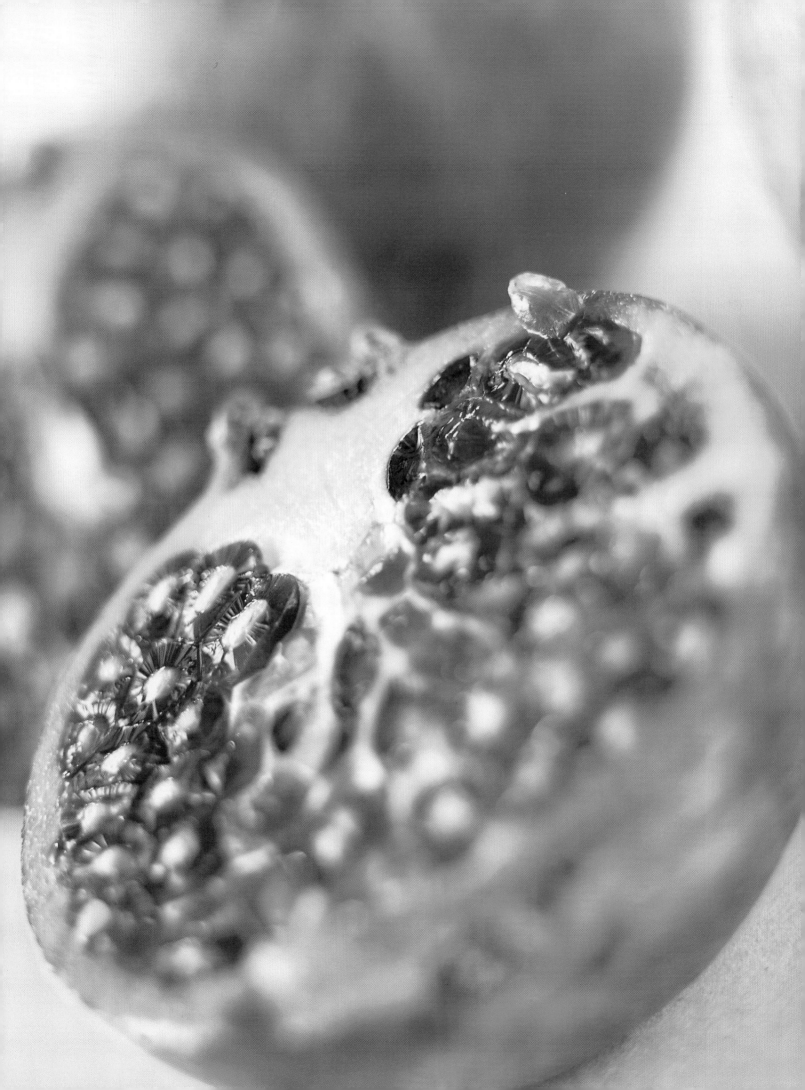

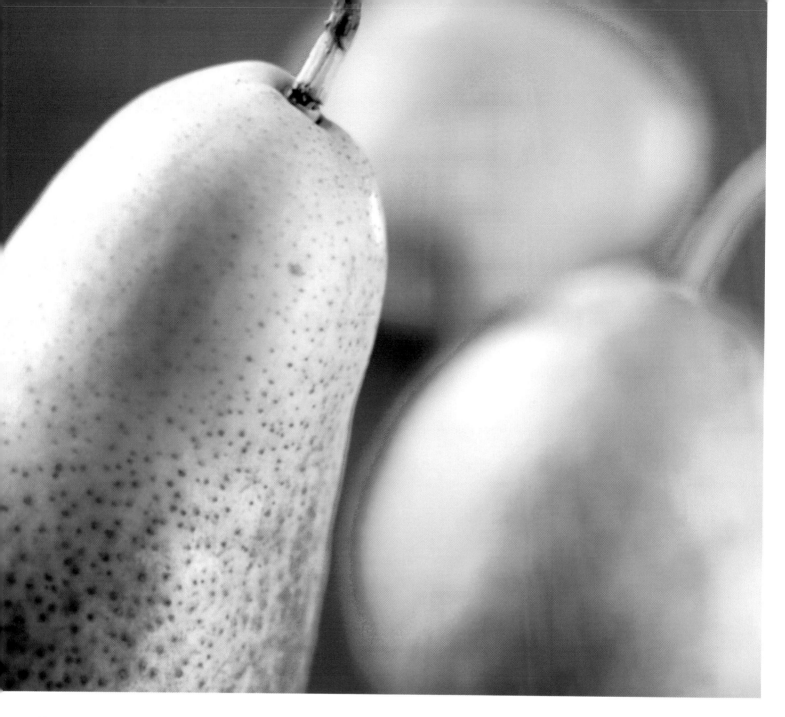

**ABOVE AND RIGHT:
PEARS AND PEACHES –
SENSUAL AND CURVY,
AS FRUIT SHOULD BE!**

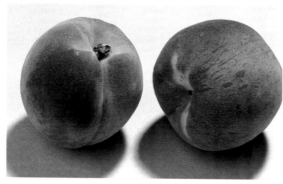

**OPPOSITE: FIGS ARE
RENOWNED THE WORLD
OVER. THEIR SECRET IS IN
THEIR HIGH POTASSIUM
CONTENT.**

make a romantic camel caravan trek across endless desert, pack dates to supply energy for the evenings under the stars!

Peaches are a luscious fruit, often linked with apricots. Their origins lie thousands of years ago in China,

where they have long been considered aphrodisiac fruits. Shakespeare, among others in history, knew of its reputation and in *A Midsummer Night's Dream* the fairies use it as an aphrodisiac. You can poach it or pickle it, but there is nothing so sensual as biting into the furry skin and silken flesh of a super-ripe peach, as messily as you can.

Pears, especially ripe pears, are popular for the same reason. Biting into their feminine roundness is very sensual. Witness the seductive dinner scene in the film Tom Jones. Their distinctive fragrance, of nail polish and boiled sweets, adds to the interest.

Figs are very suggestive fruits and their symbolism has been embraced by many nations. The Ancient Roman obscene gesture, with two fingers and a

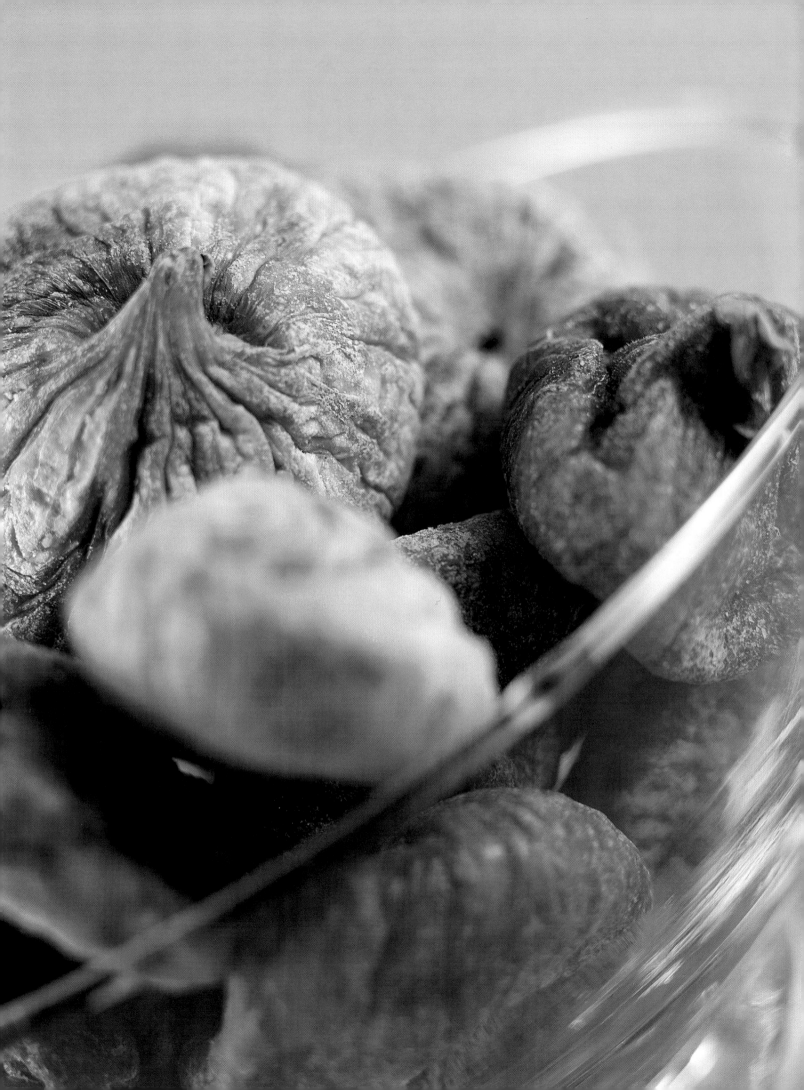

thumb, was taken up by the French, who call it 'faire le figue'. In Greece it was dedicated to love and fertility and in China it was the traditional fruit to be given to sweethearts. This has to be eaten with nature's cutlery, the fingers. Peel back the skin using only a fingernail, to reveal the sensual innards of a fresh fig. Don't buy dried ones, even in a libido-lacking emergency. The feel and look of the fig encourages lust, long before you have bitten into the flesh – the fig's, that is. As with so many of the aphrodisiacs which the ancients have handed down to us, there is a scientific explanation for the effect. In this case it is the high potassium content.

Strawberries and other berries, such as raspberries, are likened to edible pink nipples. Their eroticism is as much in their appearance and eating, as in their chemical content. Strawberries, in particular, were highly prized by Pauline Bonaparte, who produced the heir to the French empire – a feat the Empress Josephine failed to achieve. Raspberries happen to have a very high vitamin C content which may account for their effect. Strawberries are simply the epitome of luxury fruit. At fashionable sporting events in Britain, from Wimbledon to Ascot, they are *de riguer*. Try dipping them in melted chocolate, to add to the aphrodisiac result. Oddly, in classical paintings, they symbolise righteousness, as in Botticelli's *Venus and the Virgin Mary*. But don't let that put you off.

No picture of a Bacchanalian orgy is complete without satyrs and their amply proportioned partners, reclining lasciviously, dangling bunches of grapes above gaping mouths. Grapes, taken neat, do not feature largely in the history of aphrodisiacs, other than through their association with Bacchus and Dionysus. But then, they certainly consumed grapes mostly in fermented form!

Liqueurs and spirits

Before we reach the great alcoholic drinks, there are others which can aid an amorous meal. Fruit-based drinks include calvados, an apple liqueur, which is brandy-like in its silkiness. The northern French have always considered it an aid to keep youthful vigour. The Eve/apple connection sustains this belief.

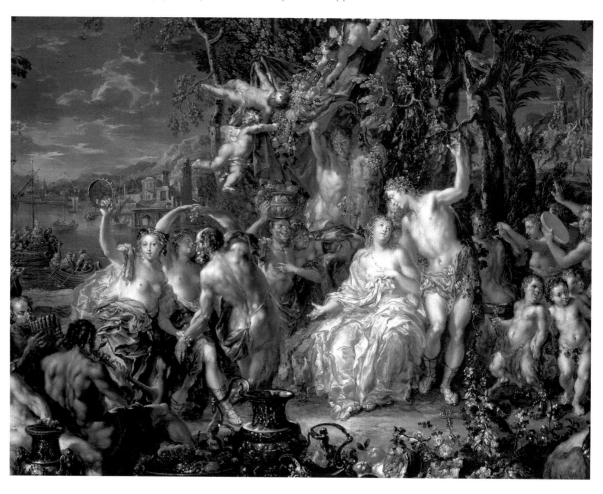

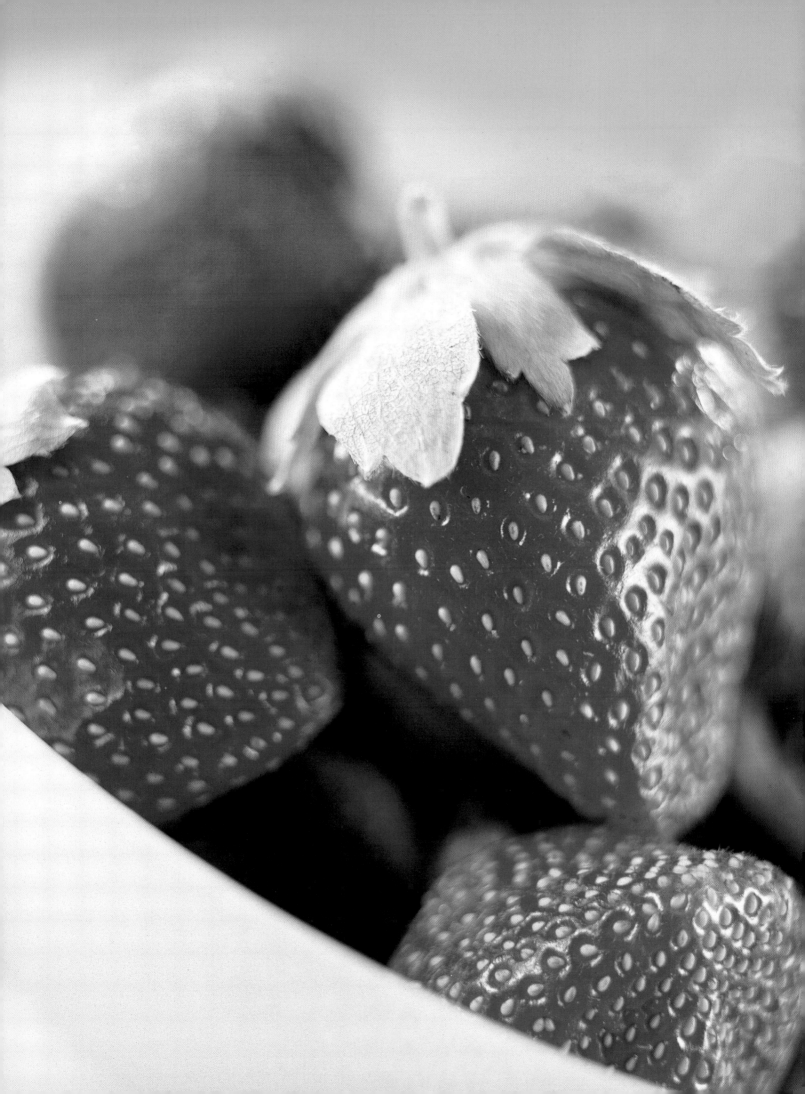

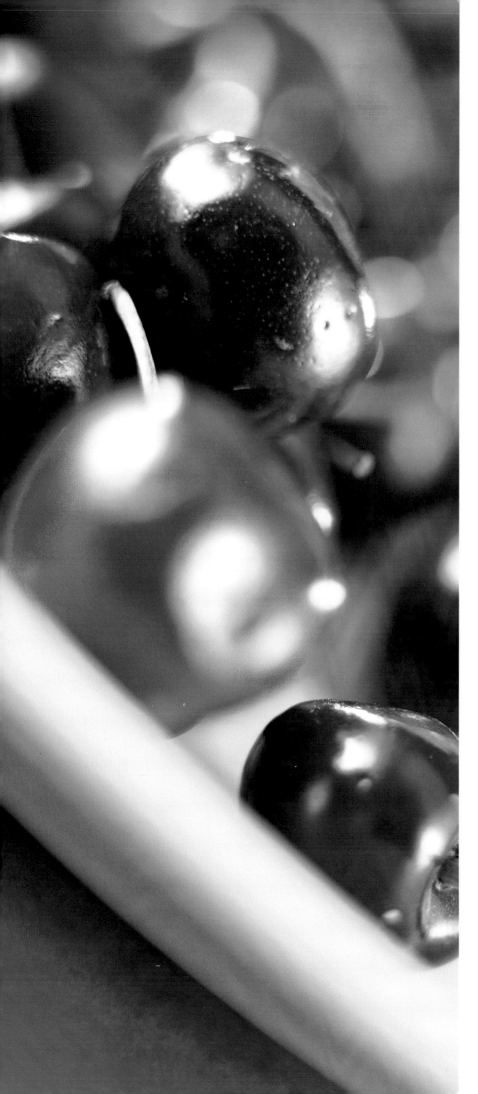

Amaretto is an Italian liqueur made from almonds, of considerable aphrodisiac force, as seen earlier when discussing the power of nuts. Kirsch is made from a fermented cherry base and gives a kick to other wines, as a mixer in cocktails or poured over fruit and ice creams. Poire Williams, a spirit made from pears of that name, is equally powerful.

Anise-based drinks have always been popular in Mediterranean countries as mentioned earlier. The French version was created by Marie Brizard in 1755 and her brand name lives on. It is the basis of several aphrodisiac drinks.

Benedictine derives its name from the order of monks who created it, not realising that they were adding to the great vat of aphrodisiacs. In Britain, the monks of Buckfast Abbey created a similar herb and honey based liqueur which has achieved notoriety, particularly in Scotland. The first two glasses are aphrodisiac because of the ingredients and quality. The following glasses (indeed, bottles) are decidedly non-aphrodisiac because of the quantity.

Another spirit to lift the libido is unadulterated vodka. The clean pure taste, allied to oysters or caviar, is unsurpassed. You do not necessarily have to take it in one shot and then smash the glass into the fireplace. But there are countless variations in vodka bars and restaurants the world over. In the Imperial Russian restaurant, Firebird, in New York, (where the decor is aphrodisiac, as well) there are over 40 different versions of vodka on offer. Their 'house' vodka brings together the aphrodisiac qualities of cinnamon, cloves, honey and cream with the vodka itself, served in an elegant flute.

Cognac and Armagnac are not in themselves particularly aphrodisiac, but they are comforting drinks to end an evening. Mundanely, they also help digestion if some over-indulgence has taken place. Port is another traditional ending to a meal, but if over-indulged by but one glass, it is likely to bring on sleepiness.

LEFT: LIFE IS JUST A BOWL OF CHERRIES.

OPPOSITE: GRAPES ARE THE PICK OF THE APHRODISIAC BUNCH.

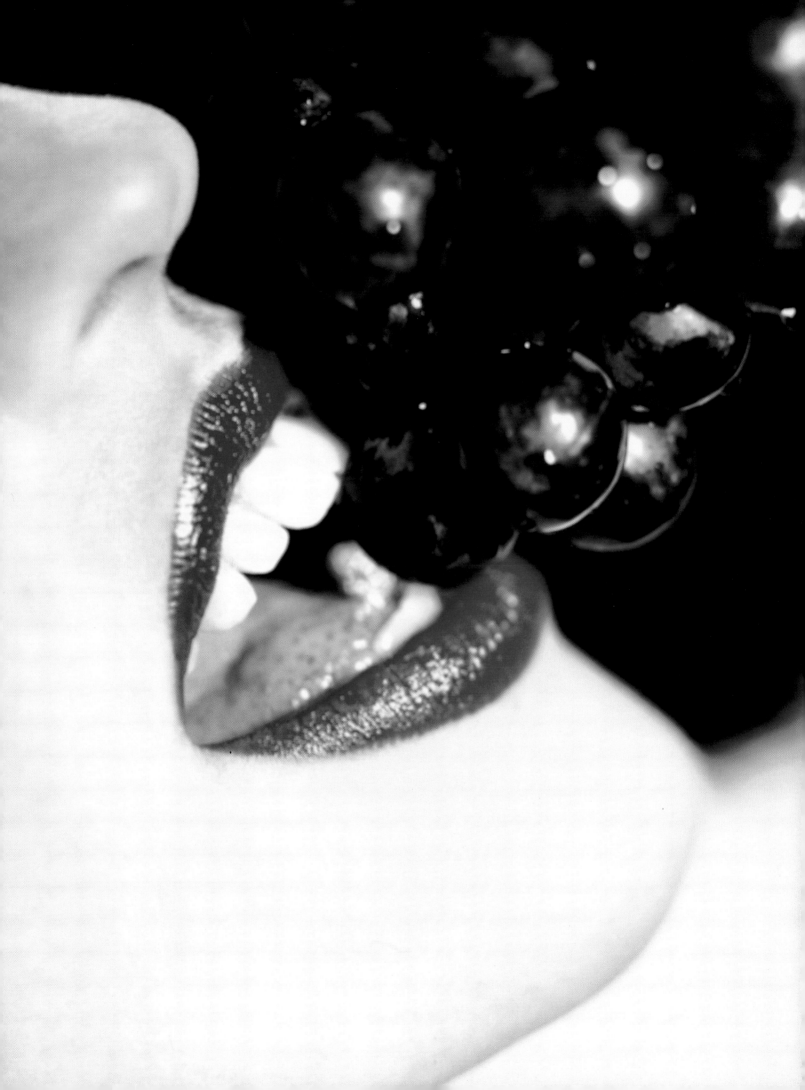

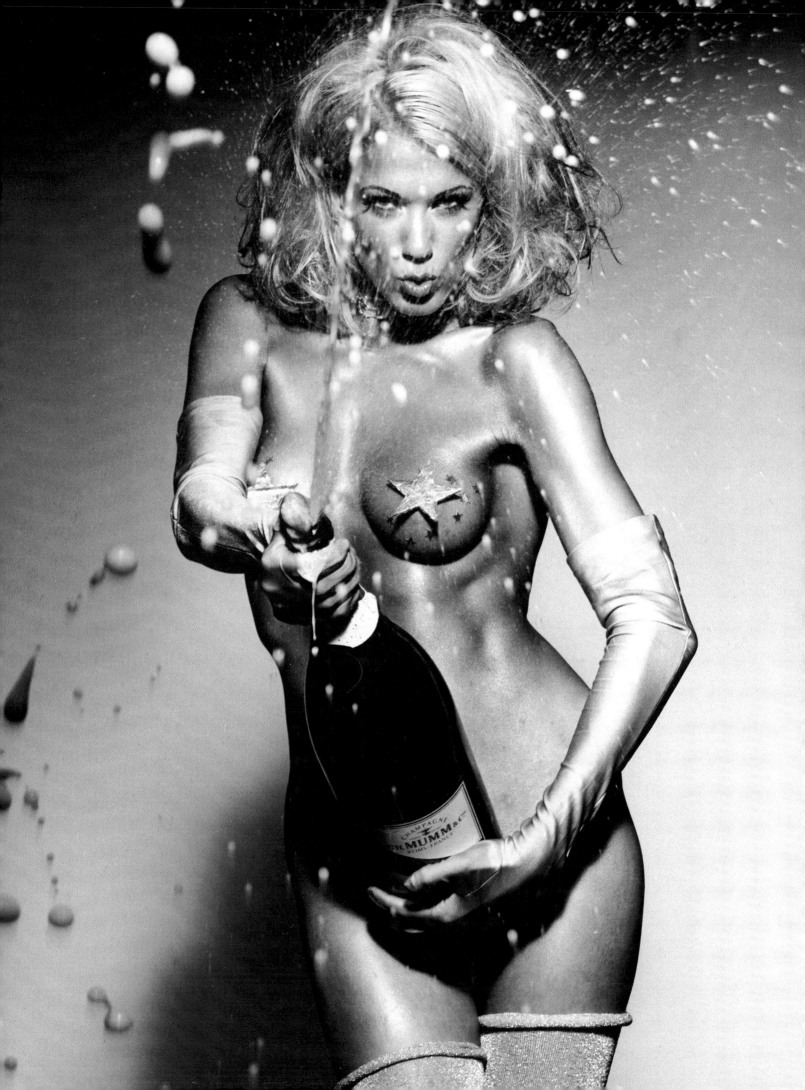

Wine and champagne

Sweet wines have long been out of fashion, but their true value is now being realised. At the turn of the century they were fashionable with aged roués, who knew their amatory importance. Their softness and roundness make the perfect end to a meal. And a single glass suffices, which is a great virtue. The emperor of sweet wines is Chateau d'Yquem, which fetches astronomical prices, thus guaranteeing its place in the aphrodisiac legend. It is invariably honey-sweet, with a gloriously aromatic bouquet.

The sweet wines of Sauternes are becoming recognised once more and can be used in a jelly to garnish foie gras, or be served cold with a ripe peach or pear after dinner. Two superior wines are Muscat Beaumes de Venise and the great Hungarian sweet, Tokay. There is also the whole range of trockenbeerenausle wines from Germany, rich sweet rieslings made from grapes which have been left to shrivel on the vines until well into winter to concentrate the juices. All have a heady bouquet which creates an amorous atmosphere.

And we come to the pinnacle of vinous aphrodisia, champagne. It is simply indispensable at any meal or other occasion when an aphrodisiac boost is needed. The pop of the cork, the rising bubbles in the glass, the burst of those bubbles in the mouth and the wonderfully uplifting taste, combine to create a truly special experience. But beware. Those very bubbles enable the alcohol to enter the bloodstream quickly, which is why the lift is quick, but it can also lead to unintentional overdrinking. Serve champagne lightly chilled so that the taste of the particular grape comes through. Too often it is much too cold. Dry, brut, champagne is the most popular, but if it is not to your taste, there are semi-sweet and sweet types available. For that very special occasion go for the greats; Roederer Cristal, Dom Perignon, Bollinger, Krug or Taittinger. But as these are truly expensive (prices will start around £60 [$100] a bottle), you may have to settle for one of the lesser champagnes, such as Moët et Chandon, Mercier, Pol Roger and a host of other marques. There are now many supermarket own-brands and unrecognisable

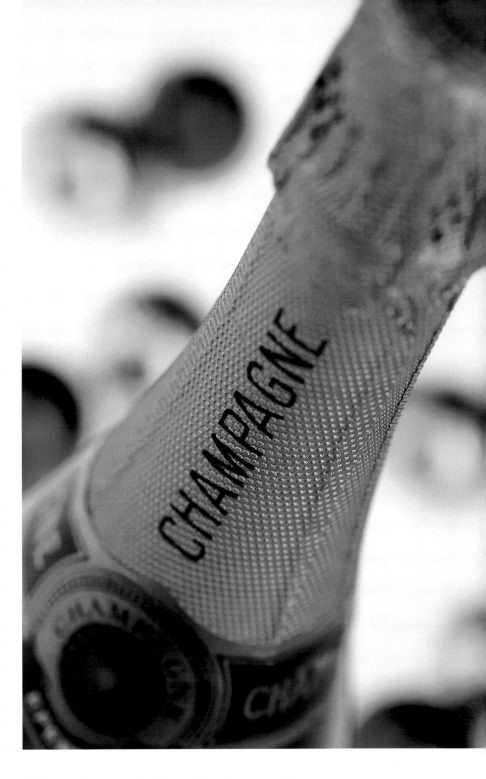

labels at the sort of price which allows you to experiment at little expense. And remember they are all champagne, the production of which is highly regulated and quality controlled.

And the perfect start or end to an aphrodisiac evening? Pink champagne. Since Prince Charles chose rosé champagne for his pre-wedding dinner, this exquisite fizz has had a well-justified renaissance. There is nothing more sensual than to enjoy the visual and spiritual experience of a flute of bubbling pink Bollinger Rosé.

OPPOSITE AND ABOVE: EXPENSIVE, LUXURIOUS AND INTOXICATING – CHAMPAGNE IS AN APHRODISIAC EXPLOSION!

THE EVE OF ST. AGNES.

John Keats

Porphyro comes to visit his love, Madeline, and Keats uses the
metaphor of food to indicate their love-making:

And still she slept an azure-lidded sleep,
In blanched linen, smooth, and lavender'd,
While he from forth the closet brought a heap
Of candied apple, quince, and plum, and gourd;
With jellies soother than the creamy curd,
And lucent syrops, tinct with cinnamon;
Manna and dates, in argosy transferr'd
From Fez; and spiced dainties, every one,
From silken Samarcand to cedar'd Lebanon.

These delicates he heap'd with glowing hand
On golden dishes and in baskets bright
Of wreathed silver: sumptuous they stand
In the retired quiet of the night,
Filling the chilly room with perfume light.
"And now, my love, my seraph fair, awake!
"Thou art my heaven, and I thine eremite:
"Open thine eyes, for meek St. Agnes' sake,
"Or I shall drowse beside thee, so my soul doth ache."

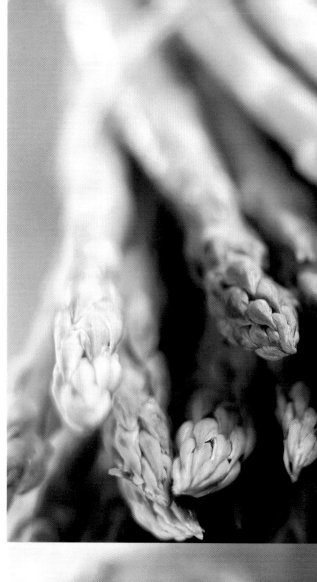

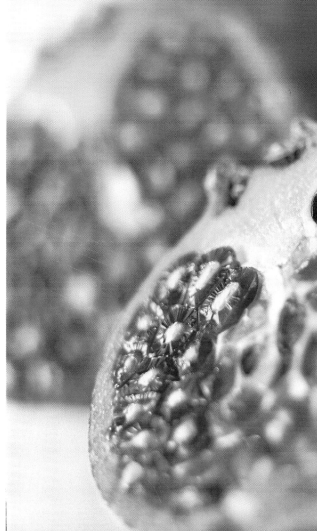

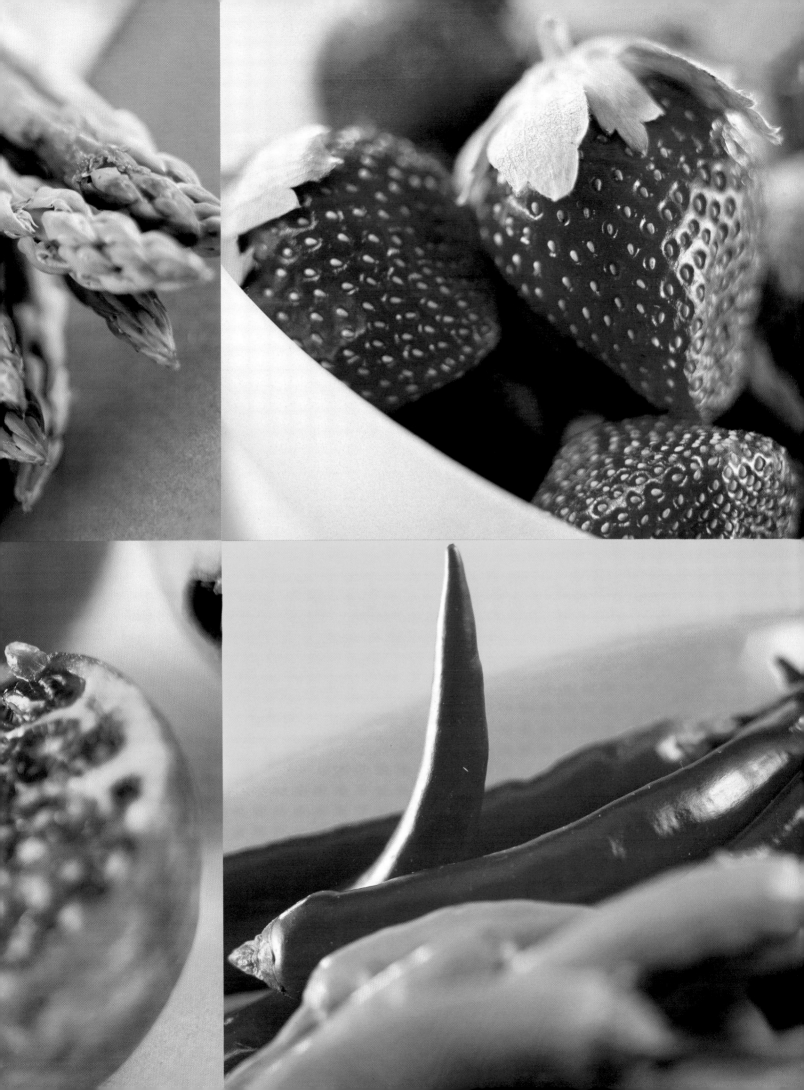

INDEX